NEUROSURGERY RESEARCH PROGRESS

NEUROENDOSCOPIC PROCEDURES AND CHALLENGES

Neurosurgery Research Progress

Additional books and e-books in this series can be found on Nova's website under the Series tab.

NEUROSURGERY RESEARCH PROGRESS

NEUROENDOSCOPIC PROCEDURES AND CHALLENGES

SONER DURU, MD
EDITOR

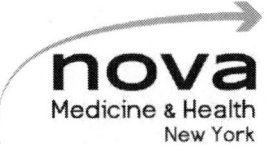

Copyright © 2021 by Nova Science Publishers, Inc.
https://doi.org/10.52305/BLPQ8705

All rights reserved. No part of this book may be reproduced, stored in a retrieval system or transmitted in any form or by any means: electronic, electrostatic, magnetic, tape, mechanical photocopying, recording or otherwise without the written permission of the Publisher.

We have partnered with Copyright Clearance Center to make it easy for you to obtain permissions to reuse content from this publication. Simply navigate to this publication's page on Nova's website and locate the "Get Permission" button below the title description. This button is linked directly to the title's permission page on copyright.com. Alternatively, you can visit copyright.com and search by title, ISBN, or ISSN.

For further questions about using the service on copyright.com, please contact:
Copyright Clearance Center
Phone: +1-(978) 750-8400   Fax: +1-(978) 750-4470   E-mail: info@copyright.com.

NOTICE TO THE READER

The Publisher has taken reasonable care in the preparation of this book, but makes no expressed or implied warranty of any kind and assumes no responsibility for any errors or omissions. No liability is assumed for incidental or consequential damages in connection with or arising out of information contained in this book. The Publisher shall not be liable for any special, consequential, or exemplary damages resulting, in whole or in part, from the readers' use of, or reliance upon, this material. Any parts of this book based on government reports are so indicated and copyright is claimed for those parts to the extent applicable to compilations of such works.

Independent verification should be sought for any data, advice or recommendations contained in this book. In addition, no responsibility is assumed by the Publisher for any injury and/or damage to persons or property arising from any methods, products, instructions, ideas or otherwise contained in this publication.

This publication is designed to provide accurate and authoritative information with regard to the subject matter covered herein. It is sold with the clear understanding that the Publisher is not engaged in rendering legal or any other professional services. If legal or any other expert assistance is required, the services of a competent person should be sought. FROM A DECLARATION OF PARTICIPANTS JOINTLY ADOPTED BY A COMMITTEE OF THE AMERICAN BAR ASSOCIATION AND A COMMITTEE OF PUBLISHERS.

Additional color graphics may be available in the e-book version of this book.

Library of Congress Cataloging-in-Publication Data

ISBN: 978-1-68507-092-2

Published by Nova Science Publishers, Inc. † New York

CONTENTS

Preface		vii
Acknowledgments		xiii
Chapter 1	The Evolution of Sympathetic Ablations from Open into Endoscopic Approaches: The Merits and Drawbacks *Moshe Hashmonai and Alan E. P. Cameron*	1
Chapter 2	How to Manage Isolated Fourth Ventricle Syndrome? *Jacintha V. Francis and M. Memet Özek*	25
Chapter 3	Radiological Evaluation of the Stoma Patency in Intraventricular Fenestrations *Aydan Arslan, Alp Dincer and M. Memet Özek*	45
Chapter 4	Endoscopic Endonasal Approach for Skull Base Pathologies in Children *Gokmen Kahilogullari*	65
Chapter 5	Endoscope–Assisted Microsurgery of Pediatric Brain Tumors *Mohamed A. El Beltagy and Mostafa M. E. Atteya*	103

Chapter 6	Suprasellar Arachnoid Cysts: Retrospective Series and Literature Review *E. Marcati, G. L. Gribaudi, M. Cenzato and G. Talamonti*	**119**
Chapter 7	Neuroendoscopic Challenges in the Treatment of Ventricular Tumors *Piero Andrea Oppido*	**147**
Editor's Contact Information		**161**
Index		**163**

PREFACE

In 1910, L'Espinasse performed the first neurosurgical endoscopic procedure for choroid plexus electrocoagulation in an infant with hydrocephalus, by use of a cystoscope. One infant was successfully treated. Walter Dandy used an endoscope to perform an unsuccessful choroid plexectomy in 1922. The next year, Mixter, using a urethroscope, performed the first successful endoscopic third ventriculostomy in a 9-month-old girl with obstructive hydrocephalus. In 1935, Scarff reported his initial results about endoscopic third ventriculostomy using a novel endoscope. His ventriculoscope had an irrigation system to prevent intraventricular collapse and was equipped with a flexible unipolar probe. In 1952, Nulsen and Spitz began the era of ventricular cerebrospinal fluid (CSF) shunting, marking the end of the initial era of neuroendoscopy. This dark period for neuroendoscopy continued until 1970s. However, in this period image capabilities of endoscopes improved with technological developments. In 1978, Vries demonstrated that ETVs were technically feasible using a fiberoptic endoscope to treat patients with hydrocephalus. In 1990, Jones and colleagues described a 50% shunt-free success rate for ETV in 24 patients with various forms of hydrocephalus. Four years later, the same group reported an improved success rate of 61% in a series of 103 patients. Currently, ETV is primarily used to treat obstructive hydrocephalus due to benign aqueductal stenosis or compressive periaqueductal mass lesions. Modern shunt-free success rates range from 80 to 95%.

The field of neuroendoscopy has extended beyond ventricular procedures. The endoscope is currently used for all types of neurosurgically treatable diseases such as obstructive hydrocephalus, various intraventricular lesions, hypothalamic hamartomas, craniosynostosis, skull base tumors, and spinal lesions and rare subtypes of hydrocephalus.

With the evolution of surgical techniques, endoscopy has emerged as a suitable alternative to many instances of more invasive methods. Surgeons using a neuroendoscope can perform many complex operations through very small incisions. Nowadays, neurosurgeons prefer neuroendoscopic surgery for many different lesions because of less damage to healthy tissue, low complication rate and excellent results. Neuroendoscopic surgery is a specialty within neurosurgery and requires a neurosurgeon to undergo specialized training.

In this book, the authors focused on neuroendoscopic procedures and challenges. The authors have created this book with the hope that it can be a guide for neurosurgeons who are interested in neuroendoscopic interventions.

Chapter 1 - Surgery of the sympathetic system evolved in three stages: *firstly* peripheral (neck and limbs), *secondly* thoracic-abdominal by open approaches, and *finally* thoracic-abdominal by endoscopy. The peripheral approach to the system (cervical ganglia and periarterial sympathetic fibers) was largely abandoned because of its drawbacks: Horner's syndrome for the neck and poor results for the limbs. The second stage in which the thoracic and lumbar ganglia were targeted achieved good ablation but required a major surgical procedure. The most important sequel of these procedures was compensatory sweating. The advent of endoscopy substantially reduced the traumatic impact of major surgery and complications such as adhesions. The standard method of ablation also changed: instead of excision, the ganglia were electrocoagulated or the chain was simply transected by diathermy or clipped. These new methods substantially simplified the procedure. In the era of open surgery, the target for sympathetic denervation of the upper limb was the second thoracic ganglion, usually with the addition of the third and sometimes of the first ganglion. During thoracoscopy, it was serendipitously discovered that lowering the level and limiting the extent of ablation reduced the degree of compensatory sweating. However, the completeness of denervation of the limb was also reduced. Nevertheless, it was considered that this is not a major issue, as endoscopic reoperations are much easier. The proper balance between the extent and level of ablation on one hand and achievement of the target on the other is still debated. In this chapter, the literature is thoroughly reviewed.

Chapter 2 - An Isolated fourth ventricle is a form of multiloculated hydrocephalus. Anatomically, there is no connection of the fourth ventricle with the third ventricle and the basal cisterns. With the pathogenesis still obscure, the best treatment remains a conundrum. The main indication for surgical intervention is progressive dilatation of the fourth ventricle with displacement of the brainstem and clinical deterioration accordingly. Surgical options can be discussed under three main headings such as cerebrospinal fluid diversion procedures, neuroendoscopic procedures and an open surgical approach. The main aim of endoscopic procedures is the fenestration of the isolated fourth ventricle with the third ventricle. Depending on the existence of a previous shunt and third ventricle anatomy, different endoscopic approaches are available.

Chapter 3 - Intraventricular endoscopic fenestration is a popular alternative treatment method that has been increasingly used in recent years. Radiological imaging tools are very important to manage these cases during preoperative, postoperative and follow-up period. In preoperative evaluation, imaging aims to show hydrocephalus status, appropriateness of endoscopic treatment and other pathologies. Postoperative and follow-up imaging will assess the efficacy of the endoscopic fenestration, state of hydrocephalus, cyst size, and possible complications.

Chapter 4 - Endoscopic endonasal approach (EEA) has become one of the popular approaches for skull base pathologies (SBP) in children despite the challenges posed by the small size of the developing skull and the narrow endonasal corridors. This review evaluates the efficacy of EEA in the pediatric age group in view of its advantages and disadvantages. Despite the anatomy-related difficulties, the outcomes of EEA are superior owing to its high rate of success and low rate of complications, and the fact that the functional and anatomical integrities of the developing skull and nose of children can be preserved through this approach. EEA is thus an effective and safe approach for treating SBP in children.

Chapter 5 - Endoscope-assisted microsurgery (EAMS) refers to the addition of neuroendoscopy as an adjunct to ordinary open microsurgical techniques to enable closer inspection of the hidden corners of the operative field and to increase the chances of achieving better extents of safe tumor resections through augmenting their benefits and obviating the drawbacks of both techniques by simultaneous or tandem integration. This chapter sheds lights on the potential benefits of EAMS in the management of complex pediatric brain tumors in the most crucial areas of the brain and the skull base through the main major neurosurgical approaches. Technical details and precautions are also covered, giving particular attention to patient safety and complication avoidance. A special focus is directed towards handling techniques, intraoperative decision making, operative steps, chronological staging, role of the assisting surgeon, and harmony within the surgical team. EAMS is especially helpful in tumors occupying the suprasellar region, cerebello-pontine angles, and the ventricular system. There is a definitive learning curve for EAMS which could be achieved by keen practicing especially in large supratentorial intra-parenchymal surgical cavities where training on these techniques could be safer.

Chapter 6 - Suprasellar arachnoid cysts (SACs) are benign collections of cerebrospinal fluid (CSF). They are reported to amount to around 9-11% of all intracranial arachnoid cysts. Wide literature exists on their origin and pathogenesis where the majority of the authors described them as congenital lesions, due to a diverticular expansion of an abnormal membrane of Liliequist or interpeduncular cistern, which cause a partial or complete obstruction of CSF. Typically, SACs expand from the prepontine space, displacing and blocking the third ventricle and/or the aqueduct, finally causing obstructive hydrocephalus. Most of the arachnoid cysts are asymptomatic and recognized incidentally with increasing frequency since the introduction of MR imaging. Presence of clinical signs or symptoms represents the main surgical indication. The treatment of these cysts is surgical. Endoscopic surgery has been advocated as the primary treatment for SACs with hydrocephalus, superior to large craniotomy or shunting. Moreover, ventriculocystocisternotomy has been found to have a higher success rate than ventriculocystostomy. Instead, the choice of the best treatment is still unclear for SACs without associated hydrocephalus. The main classification system which divides these cysts in communicating (upper diverticulum of the diencephalic membrane, from the prepontine cistern) or non-communicating (cystic dilatation of the interpeduncular cistern) has been recently reviewed by André et al. adding the asymmetrical type 3, which expands to other subarachnoid spaces. The authors report here their series of 18 patients with SACs who were treated at their Department in a 15-year period. The authors describe the endoscopic approach and analyse the clinical and radiological follow-up. The mean follow-up was 80 months. There were no mortality and no permanent morbidity. Patients with a type 3 cyst (5.5%) required a ventriculoperitoneal shunt because of persistent hydrocephalus. The majority of patients (94.5%) clinically improved except for one who remained unchanged throughout the follow-up. Radiological results were excellent in all cases. This chapter aims to underline the importance of anatomical and pathophysiological aspects and classification systems to choose the best surgical approach for each different subtype. Adding the authors' experience, the authors agreed with other authors that there is a limited role for open surgery and they recognize as well that the gold standard for SACs is nowadays the dual endoscopic fenestration.

Chapter 7 - Neuroendoscopy is presently considered a scarcely invasive surgical approach for expanding lesions bulging into the ventricle, as a relevant tool in performing bioptic procedures, discontinuation of cystic walls or tumor removal in selected cases. Furthermore, the diffusion of neuroimaging and the accurate follow-up of brain tumor patients have more frequently allowed to document tumoral and pseudo-tumoral cystic areas causing the obstruction of cerebrospinal fluid (CSF) pathways. Neuroendoscopic procedures enable fenestration of cystic lesions, in addition to third ventriculostomy or septostomy in order to restore CSF pathways. In this study, the authors evaluate their experience regarding 96 patients affected with brain tumors arising from the wall of the third or lateral ventricle. Hydrocephalus or obstruction of CSF flow was present in all their cases. The endoscopic technique, septostomy, cystostomy, third ventriculostomy (ETV) or tumor resection were alone or simultaneously performed to control intracranial hypertension. The ETV was carried out in 68 patients with non-communicating hydrocephalus. In 6 LG astrocytoma the ETV was the only definite surgical treatment. In 20 cystic tumors, cystostomy and marsupialization into the ventricle solved a relevant mass effect with clinical intracranial hypertension syndrome. In 12 patients, neuroendoscopic relief of CSF pathways by septostomy associated with Ommaya reservoir or one catheter shunt was possible. Removal was possible in 6 colloid cysts and 5 cystic craniopharyngiomas by restoring CSF flow without other procedures. After intracranial hypertension control, in 28 malignant gliomas, 18 with metastases or leptomeningeal carcinomatosis and 6 with lymphomas were allowed to continue tumor adjuvant therapy ameliorating the quality of life. In 6 cystic central neurocytomas and 12 ependymomas subsequent microsurgical removal was achieved. Other tumors included PNET, pinealoblastoma, radionecrosis and epidermoid cyst, malignant teratoma. Neuroendoscopy was found to be safe and effective, avoiding major surgical approaches and without any relevant post-operative morbidity, due to its mininvasive characteristics and reduced complications. Based on these results and on the increasing series described in the literature, endoscopic techniques should be considered the selected approach in treating CSF obstructions by para-intraventricular tumors. This surgical procedure is not limited to relief of non-communicating hydrocephalus, but it is also useful for tumor removal or biopsies and evacuation of cystic lesions. In patients affected by malignant tumors, neuroendoscopy can be performed to control intracranial hypertension before starting adjuvant chemotherapy or radiotherapy.

ACKNOWLEDGMENTS

I would like to thank Anne Riestenberg very much for great native English editing of all chapters and preparing for publication of this book.

In: Neuroendoscopic Procedures ... ISBN: 978-1-68507-092-2
Editor: Soner Duru © 2021 Nova Science Publishers, Inc.

Chapter 1

THE EVOLUTION OF SYMPATHETIC ABLATIONS FROM OPEN INTO ENDOSCOPIC APPROACHES: THE MERITS AND DRAWBACKS

Moshe Hashmonai[1,*], *MD and Alan E. P. Cameron*[2]
[1]Faculty of Medicine, Technion - Israel Institute of Technology (Retired), Haifa, Israel
[2]Ipswich Hospital, Ipswich, UK

ABSTRACT

Surgery of the sympathetic system evolved in three stages: *firstly* peripheral (neck and limbs), *secondly* thoracic-abdominal by open approaches, and *finally* thoracic-abdominal by endoscopy. The peripheral approach to the system (cervical ganglia and periarterial sympathetic fibers) was largely abandoned because of its drawbacks: Horner's syndrome for the neck and poor results for the limbs. The second stage in which the thoracic and lumbar ganglia were targeted achieved good

---

* Corresponding Author's E-mail: hasmonai@inter.net.il.

ablation but required a major surgical procedure. The most important sequel of these procedures was compensatory sweating. The advent of endoscopy substantially reduced the traumatic impact of major surgery and complications such as adhesions. The standard method of ablation also changed: instead of excision, the ganglia were electrocoagulated or the chain was simply transected by diathermy or clipped. These new methods substantially simplified the procedure. In the era of open surgery, the target for sympathetic denervation of the upper limb was the second thoracic ganglion, usually with the addition of the third and sometimes of the first ganglion. During thoracoscopy, it was serendipitously discovered that lowering the level and limiting the extent of ablation reduced the degree of compensatory sweating. However, the completeness of denervation of the limb was also reduced. Nevertheless, it was considered that this is not a major issue, as endoscopic reoperations are much easier. The proper balance between the extent and level of ablation on one hand and achievement of the target on the other is still debated.

In this chapter, the literature is thoroughly reviewed.

INTRODUCTION

Sympathetic surgery evolved in three stages: peripheral target sites (cervical ganglia and periarterial stripping in the limbs), open central procedures (thoracic and abdominal ganglionectomies), and endoscopic ablations of the same ganglia. The first stage was abandoned because of its drawbacks: Horner's syndrome for cervical ganglionectomies, and inadequate results for periarterial stripping in the limb. The second stage in which ganglia of the sympathetic chain were ablated, required major operations: thoracotomies or laparotomies. In the current (third) stage, the endoscopic approach to these ganglia is associated with a much easier recovery, shorter hospital stay and speedy convalescence. In addition, reduced trauma causes fewer adhesions, making re-operations in case of failure much easier. On the other hand, resecting the ganglia endoscopically was technically more demanding, resulting in a series of alternatives such as diathermy ablation or transection of the chain, or interruption by clipping. It was also claimed that lowering the level and limiting the extent of ganglionic ablation reduced the severity of compensatory sweating. Thus, a plethora of variations in the technique of ablation was introduced aiming to technically facilitate the procedures and reduce the consequences. Despite these achievements, controversies still exist [1].

The purpose of this chapter is to review the literature and summarize the data on the evolution of sympathetic surgery from peripheral into open central procedures, subsequently the transition into endoscopic operations, and finally the present state of art.

First Stage of Sympathetic Surgery - Historical Landmarks

It was Claude Bernard, who in 1852 provided the first major physiological understanding of the sympathetic system, namely the effect on the eye and lids (later named the Horner's syndrome) and vasodilatation [2]. Vasodilatation was further confirmed in 1879 by the experiments of Gaskell [3]. Based on the evidence that sympathetic ablation resulted in peripheral vasodilatation, the first clinical operation on the sympathetic system was performed by Alexander in 1889 [4]. He resected cervical ganglia in the neck intending to treat epilepsy. Its use was extended for the treatment of several other indications, some of them obsolete (glaucoma, "idiotie" [5], exophthalmic goiter [6], migraine [7]), some others still in use (angina [8] and hyperhidrosis [9]). In 1899, Jaboulay achieved sympathetic denervation of the lower limb by periarterial stripping to treat ischemic ulcers [10]. The procedure was extensively used and extended to Raynaud's phenomenon by Leriche [11] and by Brüning [12] for scleroderma as well.

Transition into Open Thoracic/Abdominal Operations

Historical Notes

Peripheral sympathetic ablations had two drawbacks: Horner's syndrome for cervical ablations and a high rate of inadequate results for periarterial ablations which was attributed to insufficient denervation [13]. Royle ND [14] introduced ramisectomy of the lumbar ganglia in the treatment of spasticity. He performed the first procedure on the 1st September 1923. Diez [15] extended its indication to ischemic pathologies of the lower limbs and performed the first lumbar ganglionectomy the 24th July 1924 for "syphilitic endarteritis obliterans." Adson at the Mayo Clinic initially performed lumbar sympathetic ramisectomy for spastic paralysis. Subsequently, he performed sympathectomies instead of ramisectomies. Based on his meticulous pathophysiological observations, he extended the procedures to Raynaud's disease/phenomenon [16], thromboangiitis obliterans [17] and hyperhidrosis [18] in the legs. He also introduced thoracic ganglionectomies for the same indications in the arms [19].

General Considerations

For pathologies in the upper limbs and face, the transition resulted in two major achievements. It was realized that to obtain complete sympathetic denervation of the face and upper limb, the second thoracic ganglion should be the target level [20, 21]. The target ganglia were removed thus allowing histologic examination and if in doubt, a frozen section during the operation provided confirmation. Complete sympathetic denervation was thus obtained in a high proportion of cases [22]. Failures became rare and were attributed to sympathetic fibers bypassing the sympathetic trunk (so called nerve of Kuntz) [23]. Horner's syndrome, an inevitable result of stellate ganglionectomy, simply became a rare complication of thoracic ganglionectomies [24].

Thoracic Procedures

For upper thoracic ganglionectomies, four surgical approaches were developed [25].

1. The dorsal approach: This was the first method used. The first description of the technique was published by Adson and Brown [26] in 1929. Later, it was modified by White et al. [27] and Smithwick [28]. It comprised in paravertebral muscle splitting and

rib resection. This approach allowed resection of the root ganglia together with the sympathetic trunk and ganglia. It could be performed bilaterally at the same sitting.
2. The supraclavicular approach: Telford [29] published the first description of this technique in 1935. Through a medial supraclavicular skin incision the clavicular portion of the sternocleidomastoid muscle, the anterior scalene muscle and the thyrocervical trunk artery were divided. Care was necessary to avoid injury to the internal jugular vein, the phrenic nerve, and the subclavian artery. Lastly, the Sibson's fascia is opened and the pleura is separated and retracted anterioly, exposing the sympathetic ganglia over the heads of the ribs, starting by the stellate ganglion. Simultaneous bilateral sympathectomy could be performed by two surgical teams thus shortening the operating time [25].
3. The axillary transthoracic approach: Atkins described and published this method in 1949 [30], reporting that it was devised by Schultz and Goetz [31]. A small thoracotomy was performed in the axilla, with an incision running from the pectoralis major muscle anteriorly to the latissimus dorsi posteriorly. The long thoracic nerve was safeguarded. The intercostal muscles were incised either at the level of the second intercostal space [30] or lower down in the third or fourth space [32]. The stellate ganglion or at least its cervical component was outside the surgical field, which further reduced the incidence of Horner's syndrome. Bilateral sympathectomy by this method was usually a staged procedure.
4. The anterior transthoracic approach: First suggested by Goetz and Marr [21], it was later supported by Palumbo in 1956 [33]. It employed a thoracotomy through the first, second, or third anterior intercostal space, commencing at the sternal margin. The pectoralis major muscle was split and the intercostal muscles were incised. Except for the site of the incision, this approach was equivalent to the transaxillary method. Comparison of these approaches: The

dorsal and the supraclavicular are extrapleural approaches. The first was rather aggressive, requiring removal of paravertebral rib sections, and involving a difficult convalescence. Furthermore, exposing the root ganglia as well as the sympathetic chain is not an important advantage as targeting the latter is sufficient. Therefore, the supraclavicular technique remained the preferred extrapleural approach. The other two approaches required a thoracotomy. Of the two, the transaxillary method was the most popular, the scar being less prominent and major chest muscles unaffected. Consequently, either the supraclavicular or the transaxillary approach was used, according to the surgeon's preference. The supraclavicular approach was technically much more demanding. On the other hand, it could be performed bilaterally, even simultaneously, and recovery was more rapid. The transaxillary approach was a much easier technique. However, it invaded the pleura, and was rarely performed bilaterally as a one stage procedure. Are the open procedures obsolete? With the advent of endoscopy, publications referring to the open approaches practically disappeared. However it is important that a surgeon should be able to proceed rapidly to an open approach if complications occur. For example, air embolism is a possible complication during thoracoscopy and two such cases have been published. In the first [34], sudden death occurred after division of pleural adhesions. In the second case [35], a sudden drop in end-tidal CO_2 accompanied by severe bradycardia and hypotension occurred while pneumothorax was obtained, before any dissection was commenced. This patient recovered and latter sympathectomy was performed by the supraclavicular approach. An open approach may still be required in cases with extensive severe pleural adhesions such as in apical TB.

Abdominal Procedures

Royle [14] performed the first lumbar sympathetic ablation by a postero-lateral muscle cutting extraperitoneal approach. In 1932, Adson reported a transperitoneal approach, allowing bilateral sympathectomy if required [19]. Later, in 1935 an anterior muscle splitting extraperitonal approach was described by Flothow [36] and finally adopted by Pearl after investigating three muscle splitting methods on cadavers [37]. The range of ablation varied enormously: from complete resection of the lumbosacral chain as suggested by Diez [15] to a simple division of the chain at L3-L4 or L4-L5 level as reported by Atlas [38].

Transition into Endoscopic Operations

Historical Notes

The first endoscopic thoracic sympathetic ablation was performed by Hughes in 1939 and reported in 1942 [39]. Independently, Goetz and Marr [21] described the thoracoscopic approach for the ablation of the second thoracic ganglion. However, the first large series of thoracoscopic operations for various indications was published by E. Kux in 1951 [40]. M. Kux [41] reported the first large series of thoracoscopic sympathetic ablations for hyperhidrosis in 1978. However, it is due to Drott and Claes [42] that thoracoscopy was universally established as the gold standard approach for this procedure in 1993. Widespread interest in the approach was followed by the establishment of the International Society of Sympathetic Surgery in 2001 and its biannual International Symposia.

Open surgery on the lumbar sympathetic chain was supplanted by endoscopy much later. Soderstrom initially reported the intraperitoneal approach in 1975 [43]. After an initial experimental study on pigs [44], the retroperitoneal approach was applied to humans, becoming the standard procedure for lumbar sympathetic ablation [45].

Conceptual Changes in the Operative Procedures

Endoscopy simplified the operative procedures, and recovery became shorter. In case of failure, reoperation became easier. In the open era, the second thoracic ganglion was the target for sympathetic denervation of the upper limb. This concept was validated by a human study which showed that in more than 90% of cases, the uppermost sympathetic preganglionic outflow to the hand originated in the second thoracic spinal segment (T_2) [46]. Operative success was obtaining dry hands and persisting sweating was a failure. During the endoscopic era, it was noted that when lower ganglia were targeted palmar sweating was reduced but not necessarily eliminated. This even led some authors to consider total palmar anhidrosis an undesirable result [47]. When such residual dampness became acceptable, assessment of success became problematic, raising the question: how much persisting moisture is needed and how is this evaluated? Instead of using metrics to establish what normal moisture is and to measure the residual amount of post-sympathectomy sweating, evaluation became based on the subjective satisfaction of the patient [48]. It was also claimed that the occurrence of compensatory sweating, the main untoward side-effect of the procedure, was reduced by lowering the level and restricting the number of ganglionic ablation [49]. These conceptual changes led to many modifications of the surgical procedure: at least forty two different methods were identified in one review [50].

Present Indications

Most of the early indications at the beginning of sympathetic surgery have fallen into oblivion. Ischemic disease of the limbs, which was the foremost indication in the middle of the twentieth century, could be treated by vascular reconstructive surgery in the majority of cases. In a recent review [51], the present indications were thoroughly reviewed. But since its publication, an additional indication which fell into disuse - tinnitus [52] has reappeared! [53]. Today, primary hyperhidrosis is certainly the indication for the majority of sympathetic ablations.

Techniques of Access

For the thoracic sympathetic chain, ports are introduced through intercostal spaces in a variety of locations and sites and trocar dimensions [42]. One port can be used if the telescope contains additional channels for the instruments [41], although this may restrict maneuvering. Three ports allow a separate insertion of the scope leaving the other two for bimanual use of instruments [54]. Alternatively even excision of the ganglia may be performed with a single instrument reducing the number of ports to two [55]. One or two ports remain the present standard. Apparently for cosmetic reasons, a transabdominal approach has been reported [56]. It uses a single port in the umbilicus, peritoneal insufflation, perforation of each diaphragm and bilateral pleural insufflation using a long flexible pediatric endoscope with an additional channel for instruments. Whether the benefit of a single hidden cutaneous scar overweighs the extent of the procedure is debatable [57]. Nevertheless, this technique has been used with apparent success in humans [58]. In the pursuit of a cutaneous scarless operation, an experimental study on pigs proved that a transesophageal bilateral approach to the sympathetic chain is feasible [59]. The merits of no scar must be set against the risks of perforating the esophagus and contaminating the mediastinum. It is therefore highly improbable that this technique will ever be used in humans. Recently, robotic instrumentation has been employed and claimed to improve visualization [60].

For lumbar sympathetic ablation, two techniques are in use: intraperitoneal [43] or extraperitoneal [45].

Methods of Ablation

In the open surgery era, excision of sympathetic ganglia was the standard procedure. The use of a single endoscopic instrument made dissection and excision of ganglia technically demanding and it was easier to use diathermy to thermocut the white and gray rami communicantes [41], or to coagulate the ganglia [61]. The neural sympathetic pathways to the upper limb ascend from the thoracic chain, via the stellate ganglion and ablation of the stellate (lower cervical) ganglion results in sympathetic denervation of the upper limb [62, 63]. Therefore, transecting the sympathetic chain at any level will eliminate the sympathetic supply of the upper limb originating from the truncal segment of the transection and lower down. However, some sympathetic fibers bypassing the chain [so called nerve of Kuntz] remain [23]. Anatomical transection was obtained by diathermy [61] and functional interruption by clipping [64]. Lasers and radiofrequency devices were also used to obtain ablation [65] but did not become popular. Finally, use of the harmonic scalpel [66] avoided intrathoracic smoke formation, a handicap of diathermy.

Level and Extent of Ablation

This is still the most debatable topic of sympathetic surgery. Evaluation and comparison of reports is complicated because some authors report the level of ablation by rib count -(R), others by root/trunk level (T), and finally some reports are based on ganglion count (G). The correct method should be by ganglion count because the enormous anatomical variability of the upper thoracic chain [67, 68], makes the R and T methods of reporting inadequate. Rib count is even more problematic. Satyapal et al. [69] claimed that the first rib is not visible during thoracoscopy. Contrarily, in another cadaveric study, Wong was able to see the first rib from inside the chest in half of the cases and this rib was palpable in the remaining [70].

In the first period of endothoracic sympathectomies, G_2 was the target level. However, Lin found that hyperhidrosis of the hands was reduced when the level of his procedure was lower than intended [71]. Based on this observation, he suggested that lowering the level of ablation to G_3 and later to G_4 still achieved what he conceived adequate denervation [71]. Thus, the axiom that the G_2 ganglion is the target for sympathetic denervation of the upper limb was progressively abandoned, and lowering the level and reducing the extent of ablation to a single ganglion became acceptable and adopted by the majority of authors [49, 72]. This principle was considered to lower the incidence and degree of compensatory sweating, but at the same time, some degree of palmar perspiration persisted. Thus, palmar anhydrosis was no longer considered the goal of the operation, instead it was reduction in the amount of perspiration to levels satisfying the patient [72]. An attempted "consensus" on the matter was published in 2011 [73], suggesting limiting the ablation for palmar hyperhidrosis to a transection of the chain over the third rib and considering transection over the fourth rib also acceptable. For palmar-axillary, palmar-axillary-plantar, and axillary hyperhidrosis alone, transection of the chain over the fourth and fifth ribs was advised. For craniofacial hyperhidrosis only, transection of the chain over the second and third rib was recommended. This "Consensus", however, disregarded previous observations in which limiting T2-T3 to T2-only sympathetic ablation did not reduce the amount of compensatory sweating [74], or other reports such as that of Duarte and Kux [75], in which a very extensive ablation also resulted in very low compensatory hyperhidrosis. Equally, a recent controlled trial [76] did not support the concept that lowering the level of sympathetic ablation affected the incidence or severity of compensatory hyperhidrosis. Another study, comparing T2-T3 to T2-T6 resections obtained similar results [77]. Finally, a review of the literature [50] did not support the claim that lowering the level, restricting the number of ablated ganglia or substituting resection by other methods of ablation result in less compensatory hyperhidrosis, thus, further questioning the "Consensus." In conclusion, at present, controversy persists [1]. Nevertheless, it should be stated that the majority of studies and authors favor lowering the level and limiting the number of ablated ganglia in order to reduce the occurrence and amount of compensatory hyperhidrosis at the expense of residual perspiration and increased recurrences.

Complications and Sequels

Some complications have been reduced by the change into endoscopic and mainly thoracoscopic surgery. Horner's syndrome is rarely reported, the cervical portion of the stellate ganglion being always extra thoracically located. It may be due to dissipation of diathermy heat and so can easily be totally avoided by transecting the chain at the uppermost level with clips or scissors. Pneumothorax may occur especially in the presence of adhesions and may require drainage. Bleeding may occur due to damage to intercostal vessels, anatomical variation [presence of an azygos vein], or perforation of the aorta or subclavian artery. Fatalities have not been directly reported in the literature but the authors are aware of mortality due to perforation of the subclavian artery [24] or the aorta (case mentioned at the first International Symposium on Sympathetic Surgery in 1993).

The consequences of sympathetic surgery were not altered by the transition into endoscopy. The most troublesome remains compensatory sweating, present not only when the procedure is performed for all indications, including painful syndromes [78], Raynaud's phenomenon [79], ischemic indications [80], and facial blushing [81]. During the endoscopic era two methods of reversal were introduced: removal of clips [64] and nerve reconstruction [82], intending to reduce compensatory sweating by renewed sympathetic activity to the limbs.

Reversibility by Unclipping and Reconstructions

Three animal studies examined the value of unclipping to renew the sympathetic input to the limb. Two of them excluded [83, 84] reversibility, while a later one raised the possibility [85]. However, these studies are based on histological examinations. They did not refute or confirm functional activity. Several clinical studies report reduction of compensatory hyperhidrosis as result of unclipping, not necessarily in parallel with resumed sweating. A recent thorough review of the subject [86] has concluded that early removal of the clip may allow reversibility, but insufficient evidence is available regarding late unclipping.

Reconstruction by nerve grafting was suggested by Telaranta [82]. Sporadic reports claimed some degree of reversibility by this procedure [87]. A recent report of three cases with robotic nerve graft reconstructions with detailed observations and recording of data [88], showed improvement of cardiac rate, dissipation of fatigue in all cases and reduced compensatory sweating in two out of three.

Methods of Evaluation

At present, the accepted method of evaluating results is quality of life using several questionnaires [89-92]. However, these methods are subjective. To obtain scientifically valid evaluation, objective measurement is required. In painful conditions only subjective symptoms can be recorded, albeit by visual analogue scale. For cardiac conditions, some objective evaluation is possible by electrocardiogram. For ischemic conditions, temperature and flow measurements give objective estimations.

For hyperhidrosis, the amount of perspiration in a defined body area may be metrically evaluated. Several types of instruments and methods exist such as: sudometer, evaporimeter, skin resistance and electrical sweat activity measurement instruments, ventilation capsules, and high precision weight scales for total body perspiration measurements. Such instruments should be used under standard conditions at all stages of the study. Deplorably, there are practically no reports in which results are quantified.

Benefits and Drawbacks

Evolution from open to endoscopic sympathetic ablation simplified the surgical procedures, shortening hospitalizations, even allowing in some centers to treat cases on an ambulatory basis. If needed, reoperations became much easier, both thoracic and abdominal. Hence it was possible to limit the initial procedure since any unsatisfactory result could easily be improved by reoperation to extend the ablation. Since excision of the ganglia was technically more difficult and demanding, ablations were performed by electrocoagulation of the ganglia or transection of the chain, cutting with scissors, diathermy, or by clips. Some former complications like Horner's syndrome became rare, while new ones like pneumothorax, bleeding and even mortality due to trocar perforation of major vessels, were reported. Reducing compensatory hyperhidrosis, the main disadvantage of sympathetic ablation, became a desired goal, leading to lowering the level and extent of ablation. One consequence of this approach was that totally dry hands were no longer considered the goal of surgery for hyperhidrosis and a certain amount of humidity became acceptable. The present problem is to determine how much residual humidity is acceptable and how to secure that result. Simple patient satisfaction may not be an adequate criterion as it can be distorted by "commercial" pressures, and is not "scientifically" based.

Future Perspectives

The present controversies arise because of the difficulty of retrieving valuable data from the literature [93]. To obtain scientifically based decisions, a conceptual change is required. Results should be evaluated by measurement and not solely by patient's satisfaction. Controlled trials with specific targets to be examined are required. The level of ablation should be anatomically decided by ganglion and not by rib or segment count. This is of utmost importance because of the variability of the anatomy [67, 68]. Collected data should include pictures of each procedure to allow objective evaluation by a reviewer. The exact method of ablation should be specified in the study design and meticulously observed. Pre and postoperative observations should be scientifically measured. Such criteria will also allow comparison of results obtained in various studies.

CONCLUSION

Surgery of the sympathetic system has evolved since its introduction in 1889. Early indications became obsolete and at present hyperhidrosis is the most important. The advent of endoscopy simplified the surgical procedures, shortened operating time, and allowed a more rapid convalescence. Some complications, mainly Horner's syndrome, became a rare event, while others like perforation of major vessels emerged. Compensatory hyperhidrosis has remained the most untoward sequel occurring after operations for any indication. It was serendipitously noticed that lowering the level of ablation reduced the incidence and degree of compensatory sweating, at the expense of residual moisture in the limb and increased recurrence. Although studies have been published refuting this concept, the trend to lower the level of ablation and restrict the number of ablated ganglia is accepted by the majority of authors. Endoscopic operations being easier than the open surgical procedures, resulted in reduced fear of failure. For vascular and cardiac indications, results may be objectively evaluated. For hyperhidrosis, the lack of definition regarding the right amount of acceptable residual moisture, prompted evaluation of results by "patient satisfaction." Although metrics for such evaluation exist they are not used. Patient satisfaction is important but has little scientific value. Thus, controversy persists. To solve the dilemma, meticulously organized studies using objective evaluation of results are required.

REFERENCES

[1] Hashmonai, M., Cameron, A. E. P., and Cruzat, C. S. (2015). Sympathetic ablation for primary hyperhidrosis: could controversies be solved. *Prensa Med Argentina* 101:4.

[2] Bernard, C. (1852). Sur les effets de la section de la portion céphalique du grand sympathique. *C R Séances Soc Biol Fil* 4:168-170. [The effects of transecting the cervical sympathetic chain. *C R Séances Soc Biol Fil* 4:168-170.]

[3] Gaskell, W. H. (1879). Further researches on the vasomotor nerves of ordinary muscles. *J Physiol* 1:262-302, 426/3, 426/15.

[4] Alexander, W. (1889). The Treatment of Epilepsy. *Y J Pentland, Edinburgh.* 5-17.

[5] Francois-Franck, M. (1899). Signification physiologique de la résection du sympathique dans la maladie de Basedow, l'épilepsie, l'idiotie et le glaucoma. *Bull Acad Med Paris* 41:565-594. [Physiological significance of sympathetic excision in the Basedow disease, epilepsy, idiotism, and glaucoma. *Bull Acad Med Paris* 41:565-594.]

[6] Jaboulay, M. (1900). La régénération du goître extirpé dans la maladie de Basedow et la section du sympatique cervical dans cette maladie. Martin E (Ed), Chirurgie du Grand Sympatique et du Corps Thyroîde (Les Différants Goîtres). Articles originaux et observation réunis. *A. Storck & Cie, Lyon.* 3-5. [Regeneration of the excised goiter in the Basedow disease and sympathetic surgical transection in this disease. Martin E (Ed), Surgery of the sympathetic chain and the thyroid gland (The various goiters). A compilation of original articles and observations. *A. Storck & Cie, Lyon.* 3-5.]

[7] Greenwood, B. (1967). The origins of sympathectomy. *Med Hist* 11:165-169.

[8] Jonnesco, T. (1920). Angine de poitrine guérie par la résection du sympatique cervicothoracique. *Bull Acad Med Paris* 84:93-102. [Angina cured by excision of the cervicothoracic sympathetic ganglion. *Bull Acad Med Paris* 84:93-102.]

[9] Kotzareff, A. (1920). Résection partielle du tronc sympatique droit pour hyperhidrose unilatérale (régions faciale, cervicale, thoracique et brachiale droites). *Rev Med Suisse Rom* 40:111-113. [Partial excision of the right sympathetic trunk for unilateral hyperhidrosis (right facial, cervical thoracic and brachial regions). *Rev Med Suisse Rom* 40:111-113.]

[10] Jaboulay, M. (1899). Le traitement de quelques troubles trophiques du pied et de la jambe par la dénudation de l'artère fémorale et la distension des nerfs vasculaires. *Lyon Med* 91:467-468. [The treatment of some trophical lesions in the foot and the leg by denudating the femoral artery and distention of the vascular nerves. *Lyon Med* 91:467-468.]

[11] Leriche, R. (1913). De l'élongation et de la section des nerfs périvasculaires dans certains syndromes douloureux d'origine artérielle et dans quelques troubles trophiques. *Lyon Chir* 10:378-382. [On the stretching and transecting the perivascular nerves in certain painful syndromes and trophical lesions. *Lyon Chir* 10:378-382.]

[12] Brüning, F. (1923). Zur Technik der kombinierten Resectionmethode samtlicher sympathischen Nervenbahnen am Halse. *Zentralbl Chir* 5:1056-1059. [The technique of the combined resection methods of the sympathetic neural pathways in the neck. *Zentralbl Chir* 5:1056-1059.]

[13] Hashmonai, M., and Kopelman, D. (2003). History of sympathetic surgery. *Clin Auton Res* 13(Suppl. 1):1/6-1/9.

[14] Royle, N. D. (1924). A new operative procedure in the treatment of spastic paralysis and its experimental basis. *Med J Austr* 1:77-86.

[15] Diez, J. (1924). Un nuevo método de simpatectomía periférica para el tratamiento de afecciones tróficas y gangrenosas de los miembros. *Boll Soc Cir Buenos Aires* 8:792-806. [A new method of peripheral sympathectomy for the treatment of trophic and gangrenous lesions in the limbs. *Boll Soc Cir Buenos Aires* 8:792-806.]

[16] Adson, A. W. and Brown, G. E. (1925). Treatment of Raynaud's disease by lumbar ramisectomy and ganglionectomy and perivascular sympathetic neurectomy of the common iliacs. *JAMA* 84:1908-1910.

[17] Adson, A. W. and Brown, G. E. (1932). Thrombo-angiitis obliterans. Results of sympathectomy. *JAMA* 99:529-534.

[18] Adson, A. W. and Brown, G. E. (1932). Extreme hyperhidrosis of the hands and feet treated by sympathetic ganglionectomy. *Proc Staff Meet Mayo Clin* 7:394-396.

[19] Adson, A. W. and Brown, G. E. (1929). The treatment of Raynaud's disease by resection of the upper thoracic and lumbar sympathetic ganglia and trunks. *Surg Gynecol Obstet* 48:577-603.

[20] Hyndman, O. R. and Wolkin, J. (1942). Sympathectomy of the upper extremity. Evidence that only the second thoracic ganglion need be removed for complete sympathectomy. *Arch Surg* 45:145-155.

[21] Goetz, R. H. and Marr, J. A. S. (1944). The importance of the second thoracic ganglion for the sympathetic supply of the upper extremity. *Clin Proc* 3:102-114.

[22] Hashmonai, M., Kopelman, D., Klein, O. and Schein. M. (1992). Upper thoracic sympathectomy for primary palmar hyperhidrosis: long term follow-up. *Br J Surg* 79:268-271.

[23] Kuntz, A. (1927). Distribution of the sympathetic rami to the brachial plexus. Its relation to sympathectomy affecting the upper extremity. *Arch Surg* 15:871-877.

[24] Ojimba, T. A. and Cameron, A. E. (2004). Drawbacks of endoscopic thoracic sympathectomy. *Br J Surg* 91:264-269.

[25] Hashmonai, M. and Schein, M. (1994). Upper thoracic sympathectomy - open approaches. In: Paterson-Brown S, Garden J, Eds. Principles and Practice of Surgical Laparoscopy. *W B Saunders, London*. 587-603.

[26] Adson, A. W. and Brown, G. E. (1929). Raynaud's disease of the upper extremities; successful treatment by resection of the sympathetic cervicothoracic and second thoracic ganglions and the intervening trunk. *JAMA* 92:444-449.

[27] White, J. C., Smithwick, R. H., Allen, A. W. and Mixter, W. J. (1933). A new muscle splitting incision for the resection of upper thoracic ganglia. *Surg Gynecol Obstet* 56:651-657.
[28] Smithwick, R. H. (1936). Modified dorsal sympathectomy for vascular spasm (Raynaud's disease) of the upper extremity: a preliminary report. *Ann Surg* 104:339-350.
[29] Telford, E. D. (1935). The technique of sympathectomy. *Br J Surg* 23:448-450.
[30] Atkins, H. J. B. (1949). Paraxillary approach to the stellate and upper thoracic sympathetic ganglia (letter). *Lancet* 2:1152.
[31] Atkins, H. J. B. (1954). Sympathectomy by the axillary approach. *Lancet* 1:538-539.
[32] Sternberg, A., Brickman, S., Kott, I. and Reiss, S. (1982). Transaxillary thoracic sympathectomy for primary hyperhidrosis of the upper limbs. *World J Surg* 6:458-463.
[33] Palumbo, L. T. (1956). Anterior transthoracic approach for upper thoracic sympathectomy. *Arch Surg* 72:659-666.
[34] Philip, P. P. (1949). Death from cerebral air embolism during thoracoscopy. *Thorax* 4:237-242.
[35] Shpolyanski, G., Hashmonai, M., Rudin, M., Abaya, N., Kaplan, U. and Kopelman, D. (2012). Video-assisted open supraclavicular sympathectomy following air embolism. *JSLS* 16:337-339.
[36] Flothow, P. G. (1935). Anterior extraperitoneal approach to the lumbar sympathetic nerves. *Am J Surg* 29:23-25.
[37] Pearl, F. L. (1937). Muscle splitting extraperitoneal ganglionectomy. *Surg Gynecol Obstet* 5:107-112.
[38] Atlas, L. N. (1940). A modified form of lumbar sympathectomy for denervating the blood vessels of the leg and foot, anatomic considerations. *Ann Surg* 111:117-125.
[39] Hughes, J. (1942). Endothoracic sympathectomy. *Proc Roy Soc Med* 35;585-586.
[40] Kux, E. (1951). The endoscopic approach to the vegetative nervous system and its therapeutic possibilities. *Chest J* 29:139-147.

[41] Kux, M. (1978). Thoracic endoscopic sympathectomy in palmar hyperhidrosis. *Arch Surg* 113:264-266.
[42] Drott, C., Göthberg, G. and Claes, G. (1993). Endoscopic procedures of the upper-thoracic sympathetic chain. A review. *Arch Surg* 28:237-241.
[43] Soderstrom, R. M. (1975). Unusual uses of laparoscopy. *J Reprod Med* 15:77-78.
[44] Bannenberg, J. J., Hourlay, P., Meijer, D. W. and Vangertruyden, G. (1995). Retroperitoneal endoscopic lumbar sympathectomy: laboratory and clinical experience. *Endosc Surg Allied Technol* 3:16-20.
[45] Hourlay, P., Vangertruyden, G., Verduyckt, F., Trimpeneers, F. and Hendrickx, J. (1995). Endoscopic extraperitoneal lumbar sympathectomy. *Surg Endosc* 9:530-593.
[46] Ray, R. S., Hinsey, J. C. and Geohegan, W. A. (1943). Observations on the distribution of the sympathetic nerves to the pupil and upper extremity as determined by stimulation of the anterior roots in man. *Ann Surg* 118:647-655.
[47] Chang, Y. T., Li, H. P., Lee, J. Y., Lin, P. J., Lin, C. C., Kao, E. L., Chou, S. H. and Huang, M. F. (2007). Treatment of palmar hyperhidrosis: T(4) level compared with T(3) and T(2). *Ann Surg* 246:330-6.
[48] Sayeed, R. A., Nyamakye, I., Ghauri, A. S. and Poskitt, K. R. (1998). Quality of life after endoscopic sympathectomy for upper limb hyperhidrosis. *Eur J Surg* 164(Suppl. 580):30-42.
[49] Sang, H. W., Li, G. L., Xiong, P., Zhu, M. C. and Zhu, M. (2017). Optimal targeting of sympathetic chain level for treatment of palmar hyperhidrosis; an updated systematic review. *Surg Endosc* 31:4357-4369.
[50] Kopelman, D. and Hashmonai, M. (2008). The correlation between the method of sympathetic ablation for palmar hyperhidrosis and the occurrence of compensatory hyperhidrosis: a review. *World J Surg* 32:2343-2356.

[51] Hashmonai, M., Cameron, A. E. P., Licht, P., Hensman, C. and Schick, C. H. (2016). Thoracic sympathectomy: a review of current indications. *Surg Endosc* 30:1255-1269.

[52] Garnett Passe, E. R. (1951). Sympathectomy in relation to Ménière's disease, nerve deafness and tinnitus. A report on 110 cases. *Proc R Soc Med* 44:760-772.

[53] Koning, H. M., Dyrbye, B. and van Hermert, F. J. (2016). Percutaneous radiofrequency lesion of the superior cervical sympathetic ganglion in patients with tinnitus. *Pain Pract* 16:994-1000.

[54] Hashmonai, M., Kopelman, D. and Schein, M. (1994). Thoracoscopic versus open upper dorsal sympathectomy for hyperhidrosis. A prospective randomized trial. *Eur J Surg* 160(Suppl. 572):13-16.

[55] Hashmonai, M., Kopelman, D., Ehrenreich, M. and Assalia, A. (1998). The learning curve of thoracoscopic sympathectomy. *6th World Congress of Endoscopic Surgery*. Montori A, Lirici MM, Montori J, Eds. Monduzzi Editore, Bologna. 1147-1151.

[56] Zhu, L. H., Chen, L., Yang, S., Kiu, D., Zhang, J., Cheng, X. and Chen, W. (2013). Embryonic NOTES thoracic sympathectomy for palmar hyperhidrosis. Results of a novel technique and comparison with the VATS procedure. *Surg Endosc* 27:4124-4129.

[57] Hashmonai, M., Licht, P. B., Schick, C. H., Bischof, G., Cameron, A. E, Connery, C. C. and de Campos, J. R. M. (2014). Transumbilical thoracic sympathectomy with an ultrathin flexible endoscope in a series of 38 patients. (Letter to Editor) *Surg Endosc* 28:1380.

[58] Zhu, L. H., Chen, S., Chen, W., Yang, S. and Ku, Z. T. (2016). Transumbilical thoracic sympathectomy: a single center experience of 148 cases with up to 4 years of follow-up. *Eur J Cardiothorac Surg* 49(Suppl. 1):i79-i83.

[59] Turner, B. G., Gee, D. W, Cizginer, S., Konuk, Y., Karaca, C., Willingham, F., Mino-Kenudson, M., Morse, C., Rattner, D. W. and Brugge, W. R. (2011). Feasibility of endoscopic transesophageal thoracic sympathectomy (with video). *Surg Endosc* 25:913-918.

[60] Coveliers, H., Meyer, M., Gharagozloo, F., Wisselink, W., Rauwerda, J., Margolis, M., Tempesta, B. and Strother, E. (2013). Robotic selective postganglionic thoracic sympathectomy for the treatment of hyperhidrosis. *Ann Thorac Surg* 95:269-74.

[61] Lin, C. C. (1992). Extended thoracoscopic T2-sympathectomy in the treatment of hyperhidrosis: experience with 130 consecutive cases. *J Laparoendosc Surg* 2:1-6.

[62] Guttman, L. (1940). The distribution of disturbances of sweat secretion after extirpation of certain sympathetic cervical ganglia in man, *J Anat* 74:537-549.

[63] Pather, N., Partab, P., Singh, B. and Satyapal, K. S. (2006). Cervicothoracic ganglion: its clinical implication. *Clin Anat* 19:323-326.

[64] Lin, C. C., Mo, L. R., Lee, L. S., Ng, S. M. and Huang, M. H. (1998). Thoracoscopic T2-sympathetic block by clipping-a better and reversible operation for treatment of hyperhidrosis palmaris: experience with 326 cases. *Eur J Surg* 164(Suppl. 580):13-16.

[65] Massad, M., LoCicero, J. 3rd, Matano, J., Oba, J., Greene, R., Gilbert, J. and Hartz, R. (1991). Endoscopic thoracic sympathectomy: evaluation of pulsatile laser, non-pulsatile laser, and radiofrequency-generated thermocoagulation. *Lasers Surg Med* 11:18-25.

[66] Kopelman, D., Bahous, H., Assalia, A. and Hashmonai, M. (2001). Upper dorsal thoracoscopic sympathectomy for palmar hyperhidrosis. The use of harmonic scalpel versus diathermy. *Ann Chir Gynaecol* 90:203-205.

[67] Chung, I. H., Oh, C. S., Koh, K. S., Kim, H. J., Paik, H. C. and Lee, D. Y. (2002). Anatomic variations of the T_2 nerve root (including the nerve of Kuntz) and their implications for sympathectomy. *J Thorac Cardiovasc Surg* 123:498-501.

[68] Kim, D. H., Hong, Y. J., Hwang, J. J., Kim, K. D. and Lee, D. Y. (2008). Topographical considerations under video-scope guidance in the T3,4 levels sympathetic surgery. *Eur J Cardiothorac Surg* 33:786-789.

[69] Satyapal, K. S., Singh, B., Partab, P., Ramsaroop, I. and Pather, N. (2003). Thoracoscopy: a new era for surgical anatomy. *Clin Anat* 16:538-541.

[70] Wong, C. W. (1997). Transthoracic video endoscopic electrocautery of sympathetic ganglia for hyperhidrosis: special reference to localization of the first and second ribs. *Surg Neurol* 47:224-230.

[71] Lin, C. C. and Wu, H. H. (2001). Endoscopic T_4-sympathic block by clamping (ESB_4) in treatment of hyperhidrosis palmaris et axillaris - experience in 165 cases. *Ann Chir Gynaecol* 90:167-169.

[72] Hashmonai, M. (2016). The history of sympathetic surgery. *Thorac Surg Clin* 26:383-388,.

[73] Cerfolio, R. J., De Campus, J. R. M., Bryant, A. S., Connery, C. C., Miller, D. L., DeCamp, M. M, McKenna, R, J. and Krasna, M. J. (2011). The society of thoracic surgeons expert consensus for the surgical treatment of hyperhidrosis. *Ann Thorac Surg* 91:1642-1648.

[74] Licht, P. B. and Pilegaard, H. K. (2004). Severity of compensatory sweating after thoracoscopic sympathectomy. *Ann Thorac Surg* 78:427-431.

[75] Duarte, J. B. V. and Kux, P. (1998). Improvements in video-endoscopic sympathicotomy for the treatment of palmar, axillary, facial and palmar-plantar hyperhidrosis. *Eur J Surg* 164(Suppl. 580):9-11.

[76] Cai, S., Huang, S., An, J., Li, Y., Weng, Y., Liao, H., Chen, H., Liu, L., He, J. and Zhang, J. (2014). Effect of lowering or restricting sympathectomy levels on compensatory sweating. *Clin Auton Res* 24:143-149.

[77] Gunn, T. M., Davis, D. M., Speicher, J. E, Rossi, N. P., Parekh, K. R., Lynch, W. R., Iannettoni, M. D. (2014). Expended level of sympathetic chain removal does not increase the incidence or severity of compensatory hyperhidrosis after endoscopic thoracic sympathectomy. *J Thorac Cardiovasc Surg* 148;2673-2676.

[78] Bandyk, D. F., Johnson, B. L. and Kirkpatrick, A. F. (2002). Surgical sympathectomy for reflex sympathetic dystrophy syndromes. *J Vasc Surg* 35:269-277.

[79] Thune, T. H., Ladegaard, L. and Licht, P. B. (2006). Thoracoscopic sympathectomy for Raynaud's phenomenon - a long term follow-up study. *Eur J Vasc Endovasc Surg* 32:198-202.

[80] Coveliers, H., Hoexum, F., Rauwerda, J. A. and Wisselink, W. (2016). Endoscopic thoracic sympathectomy for upper limb ischemia. A 16 year follow-up in a single center. *Surgeon* 14:265-269.

[81] Girish, G., D'souza, R. E., D'souza, P., Lewis, M. G. and Baker, D. M. (2017). Role of surgical thoracic sympathetic interruption in treatment of facial blushing: s systematic review. *Postgrad Med* 129:267-275.

[82] Telaranta, T. (1998). Secondary sympathetic chain reconstruction after endoscopic thoracic sympathicotomy. *Eur J Surg* 164(Suppl. 580):17-18.

[83] Loscertales, J., Congregado, M., Jimenes-Merchan, R., Gallardo, G., Trivino, A., Moreno, S., Loscertales, B. and Galera-Ruiz, H. (2012). Sympathetic chain clipping for hyperhidrosis is not a reversible procedure. *Surg Endosc* 26:1258-1263.

[84] Candas, F., Corur, R., Haholu, A., Yiyit, N., Yildizhan, A., Gezer, S., Sen, H. and Isitmangil, T. (2012). The effect of clipping on thoracic sympathetic nerve in rabbits: early and late histopathological findings. *Thorac Cardiovasc Surg* 60:280-284.

[85] Thomsen, L. L., Mikkelsen, R. T., Derejko, M., Schrøder, H. D. and Licht, P. B. (2014). Sympathetic block by metal clips may be a reversible operation. *Interact Cardiovasc Thorac Surg.* 19:908-913.

[86] Hyes, C. F. and Marshall, M. B. (2016). Reversibility of sympathectomy for primary hyperhidrosis. *Thorac Surg Clin* 26:421-426.

[87] Haam, S. J., Park, S. Y., Paik, H. C. and Lee, D. Y. (2010). Sympathetic nerve reconstruction for compensatory hyperhidrosis after sympathetic surgery for primary hyperhidrosis. *J Korean Med Sci* 25:597-601.

[88] Connery, C. C. (2016). Reconstruction of the sympathetic chain. *Thorac Surg Clin* 26:427-434.

[89] Amir, M., Arish, A., Weinstein, Y., Pfeffer, M. and Levy, I. (2000). Impairment in quality of life among patients seeking surgery for hyperhidrosis (excessive sweating): preliminary results. *Isr J Psychiatry Relat Sci* 37:25-31.

[90] Swan, M. C. and Paes, T. (2001). Quality of life evaluation following endoscopic transthoracic sympathectomy for upper limb and facial hyperhidrosis. *Ann Chir Gynaecol* 90:177-159.

[91] De Campos, J. R. M., Kauffman, P., Werebe E. de C., Andrade Filho, L. O., Kusniek, S., Wolosker, N. and Jatene, F. B. (2003). Quality of life, before and after thoracic sympathectomy: report on 378 operated patients. *Ann Thorac Surg* 76:886-891.

[92] Delaplace, M., Dumont, P., Lorette, G., Machet, I., Lagier, I., Maruanu, A. and Samimi, M. (2015). Factors associated with long-term outcome of endoscopic thoracic sympathectomy for palmar hyperhidrosis: a questionnaire survey in a cohort of French patients. *Br J Dermatol* 172:805-807.

[93] Henteleff, H. J. and Kalavrouziotis, D. (2008). Evidence-based review of the surgical management of hyperhidrosis. *Thorac Surg Clin* 18:209-216.

Chapter 2

HOW TO MANAGE ISOLATED FOURTH VENTRICLE SYNDROME?

*Jacintha V. Francis[1] and M. Memet Özek[2],**

[1] Acıbadem University, School of Medicine, Department of Neurosurgery, Division of Pediatric Neurosurgery, İstanbul, Turkey
[2] Department of Neurosurgery, Division of Pediatric Neurosurgery, Acıbadem University, School of Medicine, İstanbul, Turkey

ABSTRACT

An Isolated fourth ventricle is a form of multiloculated hydrocephalus. Anatomically, there is no connection of the fourth ventricle with the third ventricle and the basal cisterns. With the pathogenesis still obscure, the best treatment remains a conundrum. The main indication for surgical intervention is progressive dilatation of the fourth ventricle with displacement of the brainstem and clinical deterioration accordingly. Surgical options can be discussed under three main headings such as cerebrospinal fluid diversion procedures, neuroendoscopic procedures and an open surgical approach. The main aim of endoscopic procedures is the fenestration of the isolated fourth

---

* Corresponding Author's E-mail: memetozek@gmail.com.

ventricle with the third ventricle. Depending on the existence of a previous shunt and third ventricle anatomy, different endoscopic approaches are available.

Keywords: Isolated fourth ventricle, slit ventricle syndrome, neuroendoscopy, neuronavigation

TREATMENT OF AN ISOLATED FOURTH VENTRICLE

An Isolated fourth ventricle is a form of multiloculated hydrocephalus. Anatomically there is no connection between the fourth ventricle with the third ventricle and the basal cisterns. There have been many descriptions of this entity, with 'trapped' [12] 'sequestrated' [14] 'encysted' [16] and disproportionately large fourth ventricle [24] all quoted in medical literature. In this chapter, we will be referring to this condition as the isolated fourth ventricle (IFV). In 1980, Folts et al., [5] first described IFV as being like a double compartment hydrocephalus.

Table 1. Etiologies of IFV

Post-hemorrhagic hydrocephalus
Post meningitis/ ventriculitis hydrocephalus
Dandy Walker syndrome
Over-drainage of the shunt
Radiation induced ventriculitis

It has been postulated that there is a further reduction in supratentorial intraventricular pressure, especially where there is an already low intraventricular pulse pressure and brain compliance in a shunted patient, producing a functional occlusion to the cerebral aqueduct [1]. However, the concept of having a pathologically dilated fourth ventricle, means there should be a simultaneous outlet obstruction [17]. For this to occur, another likely cause is an inflammatory process bringing about obstruction at the foramina of Luschka or foramen of Magendie, causing a morphological occlusion [1, 10]. Despite these postulations, the pathogenesis of IFV is still obscure. In addition, Montgomery et al., points out other possible etiologies that could give rise to IFV. These include Dandy Walker syndrome, slit ventricle syndrome and radiation induced ventriculitis [15] (Table 1).

CLINICAL PRESENTATION

The clinical idiosyncrasy in IFV can be conspicuous. Symptoms of IFV may be a diagnostic dilemma, especially in patients with pre-existing developmental delays and neurological deficits, and may even go undetected [13]. In our experience at Acibadem University, most of these patients are asymptomatic and sometimes detected during routine neuroimaging follow-ups.

When there is progressive dilatation of the fourth ventricle there will be compression of the adjacent neural structures, especially the cerebellum, brainstem and stretching of the exiting cranial nerves. Patients can present with a spectrum of symptomatology with initial increasing intracranial pressure symptoms such as headaches, irritability, vomiting, cerebellar instability, or even bulbar dysfunction to advanced symptoms mimicking presentation of a posterior fossa syndrome that are usually elicited by posterior fossa mass lesions [8, 16].

These signs could include cranial neuropathies due to compression of their nuclei at the floor of the fourth ventricle such as strabismus or double vision due to abducens nuclei compression, facial palsy due to facial colliculus compression and also lower cranial nerve signs such as difficulty in swallowing or tolerating feeds in a child, frequent hiccup attacks or even dysarthria. Brainstem signs include Parinaud syndrome, internuclear ophthalmoplegia, spastic paralysis of the extremities due to disruption of corticospinal tracts especially near the pontine region, gaze palsies due to compression of medial longitudinal fasciculus and pontine gaze centers, postural opisthotonos, respiratory distress or bradycardia [8].

In 1986, Cocker et al., also reported bobble-head doll syndrome in which there is intermittent anterior- posterior rhythmic bobbing of the head. This is possibly caused by the compression of the dorsomedial red nucleus due to aqueduct expansion [4]. When the reticular activating system is compressed, the patient will then have altered sensorium or eventually become comatose [8].

When a patient is symptomatic, or if there is demonstrable progression in radiological findings, the patient should be considered for surgical treatment [8].

Radiological features are principal in the diagnosis of IFV and its progression. Analysis of these imaging features could further aid in the approach and choice of surgical management. Mindful assessment of the radiological anatomy – especially of the third ventricle and its contents, cerebral aqueduct, and the basal cisterns – is crucial for planning and anatomy being favorable for endoscopic approaches.

With certain MRI sequences such as 3D CISS (three-dimensional constructive interference in the steady state) it is possible to demonstrate the presence of any membranous structure in the third ventricle or related structures near the third ventricle like adhesions such as inter-hypothalamic or interthalamic adhesions. Moreover, the size and patency of the third ventricle can be further assessed to determine the suitability of an endoscopic approach from the foramen of Monro through the third ventricle to the aqueduct [18]. At Acıbadem University, we follow this meticulous preoperative assessment of these structures to aid in our selection of patients favorable for the supratentorial endoscopic approach.

The classical radiological features of IFV explained in literature consist of an inverted funneling at the level of the aqueduct representing a stenosis with dilated fourth ventricle causing mass effect on the brainstem and cerebellum [26]. A lack of flow void in the cerebral aqueduct with a 3D CISS MRI sequence also indicates an inlet obstruction. Additionally, the demonstration of membranes dividing the cisterns and the fourth ventricle either in the foramen of Magendie or Luschka shows a fourth ventricular outlet obstruction [18].

Moreover, a vital observation elaborated upon by Udayakumar et al., [26] is the presence of diencephalic edema and transtentorial upward herniation. These findings are associated with increased pressure within the fourth ventricle.

MANAGEMENT OF IFV

Despite a variety of surgical approaches discussed in current literature, a conclusion of the best treatment for IFV remains a conundrum. Ideal as it may be, achieving the aim of having treatment with the lowest complication rate and best outcomes can be a difficult feat to accomplish.

The current established indication for surgical intervention in patients with IFV is when there is clinical deterioration and progressive dilatation of the fourth ventricle with displacement of the brainstem [13].

The surgical options described in the literature can be discussed under the following three main headings: 1) Classical CSF diversion procedures 2) Endoscopic procedures and 3) Open surgical procedures.

CSF DIVERSION PROCEDURES

The most common of these is fourth ventriculoperitoneal shunting [8]. If a functioning shunt system is present in the lateral ventricles then there are options to place a second catheter into the fourth ventricle through different trajectories, or with the aid of an endoscope [3, 13, 23]. The catheter in the fourth ventricle can then be connected to a separate distal shunt system or joined to the existing shunt system with a 'Y' connecter, either proximal or distal to the valve [3, 9, 13] (Figure 1).

The usual established routes for fourth ventricular catheter placement are via a midline transforaminal or lateral trans-cerebellar. In the transcerebellar route entry, a burr hole is made at the paramedian perpendicular to the fourth ventricular floor [13, 22]. Whereas in the midline transforaminal route, the trajectory of the catheter is perpendicular to the brainstem along its axis traversing through the foramen of Magendie to the fourth ventricle [8].

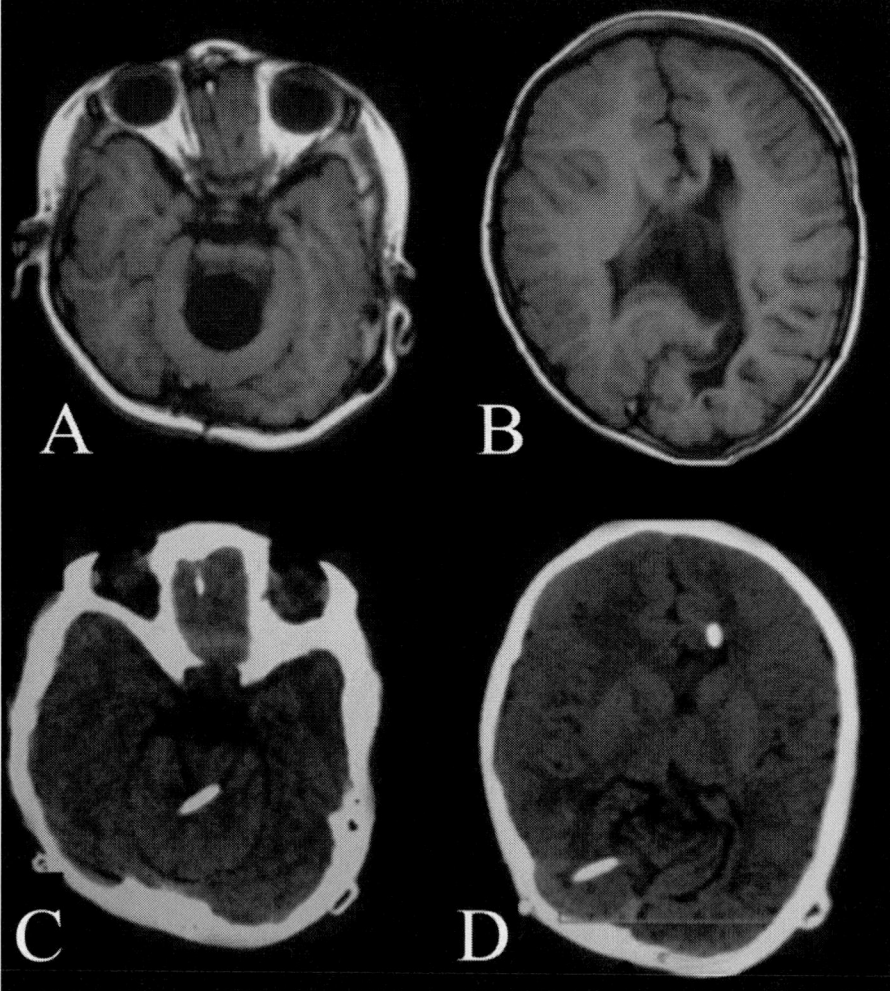

Figure 1. (A) *Preoperative* axial T1 MRI demonstrating dilated fourth ventricle. (B) Normal or non-dilated well decompressed appearance of the lateral ventricles with an existing frontal shunt. (C) and (D) Postoperative axial CT showing placement of the shunt catheter in the fourth ventricle which is now slit like and the frontal preexisting shunt in situ.

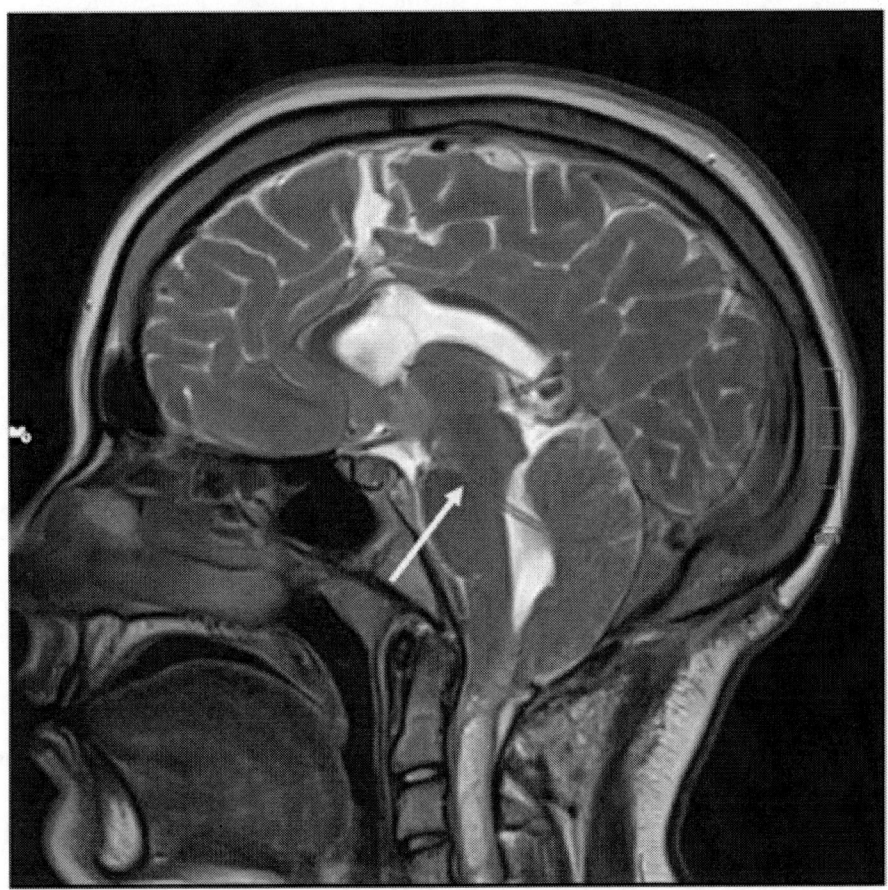

Figure 2. Sagittal T2 MRI (red arrow) showing the catheter tip penetrating the brainstem. This could be a complication of sudden decompression of the fourth ventricle and expansion of the brainstem.

Unfortunately, there were complications secondary to drastic decompression of the fourth ventricular space and expansion of the brainstem allowing it to be injured by the adjacent ventricular catheter causing neurological deficits [2, 8] (Figure 2).

Montes et al., [14] popularized the approach to the fourth ventricle through the transcortical –trans tentorial hiatus with the aid of standard stereotactic techniques locating the site of catheter site insertion and calculating precise trajectory in respect of the deep venous structures. A parietal burr hole was usually the site of entrance in the procedure (10 cm from the external protuberance and 2cm from the midline). The aim of the procedure is to equalize the transtentorial pressure and encourage CSF drainage.

ENDOSCOPIC PROCEDURES

With the emerging field of neuroendoscopy and neuroimaging, especially with the adjunct of neuro-navigation, there is now an alternative approach to IFV treatments [3, 6, 7, 8, 13, 21]. The feasibility of neuroendoscopy in aqueductoplasty and stenting was first described in detail by Shin et al., [23] in an adult patient with IFV.

Neuronavigation is an upcoming tool in most neuroendoscopic neurosurgical procedures but there is still the need for a proper selection criterion. Its usage is currently debatable with no clear consensus. Rohde et al., [18] illustrated that neuronavigation as an adjunct in intracranial endoscopic procedures is essential in only 16.7% cases, not beneficial in 43.7% and beneficial but not essential in 39.6%. Therefore, more studies are necessary for the selected cases to justify these numbers. However, in our operative setting at Acıbadem University we use neuronavigation for the treatment of IFV.

In current literature is has been well established that prerequisites for endoscopic choice of procedures in IFV are features of short segment (< 5mm) stenosis and a veil or membranous aqueduct. These are the favorable types of aqueduct stenosis that will yield good outcomes for aqueductoplasty [11, 13].

Additionally, in our centre, we divided our selection of endoscopic treatment approaches based on two main types of radiological presentation (Table 2).

Table 2.

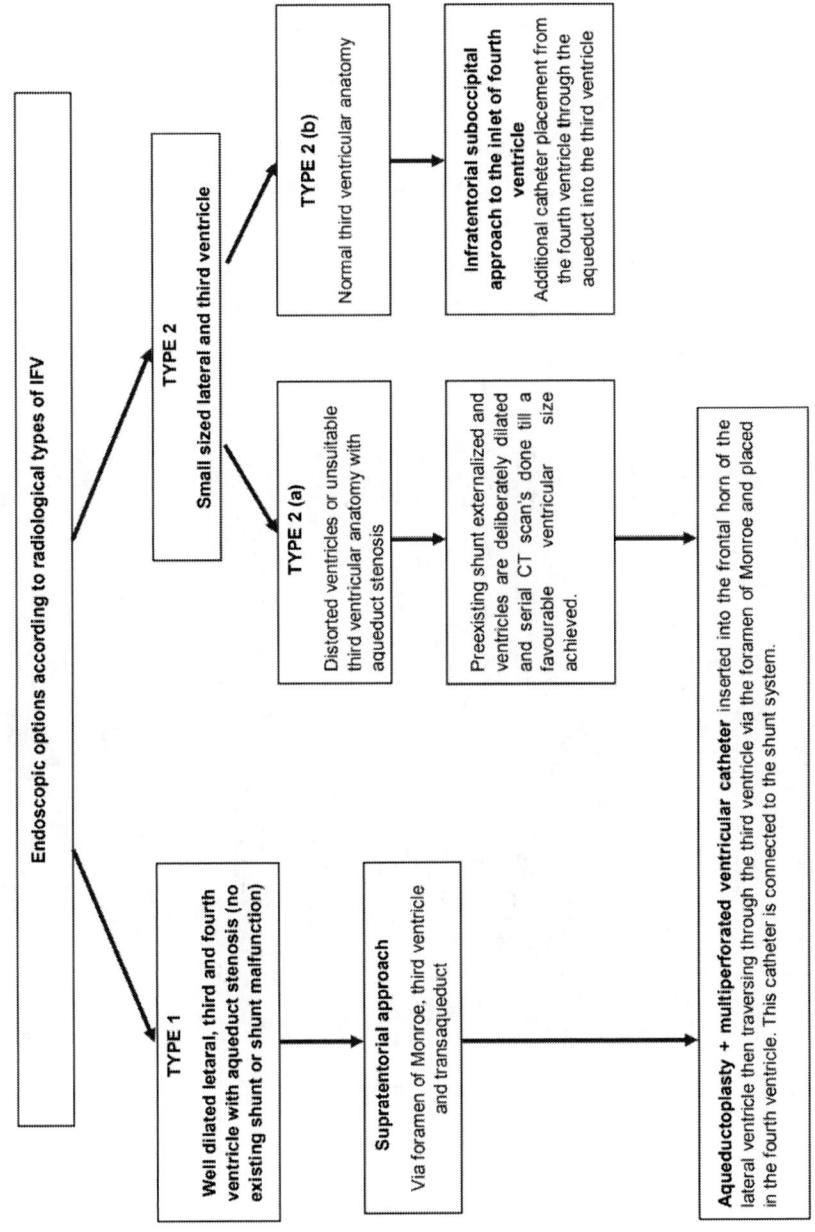

Type 1 is where there is a well-dilated lateral, third and fourth ventricle with aqueduct stenosis in patients with either no preexisting shunts or malfunctioning shunts. In these patients we attempt the supratentorial trans-third ventricle approach as described by Cinalli et al., [3] and Teo et al., [25]. A pre-coronal burr-hole is created about 4 cm anterior to the coronal suture at mid-pupillary point and an endoscope is introduced into its trajectory towards the foramen of Monroe into the third ventricle and identifying the aqueduct. A balloon catheter is inserted and the tip of the balloon is used to perforate any membrane obstructing the inlet of the aqueduct, after which the cavity of the fourth ventricle is inspected [3] (Figure 3).

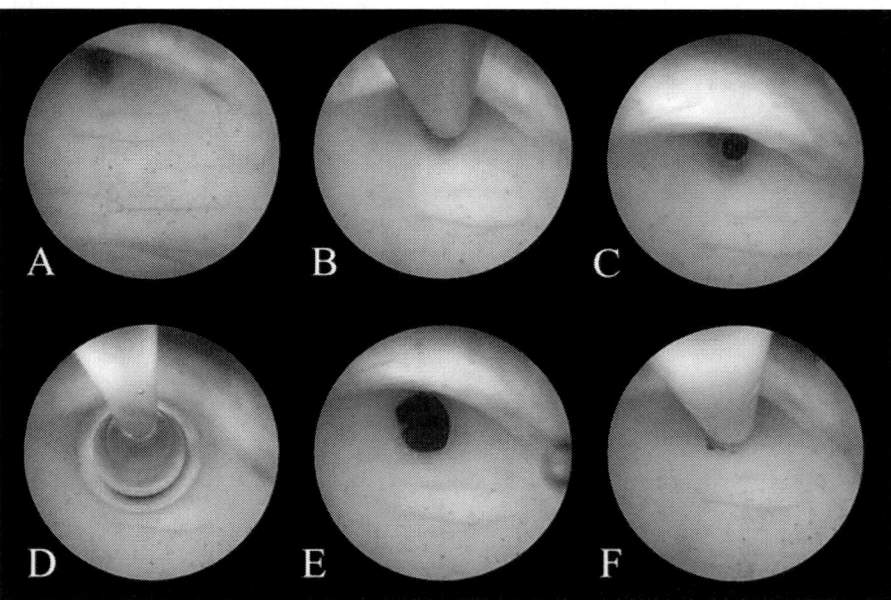

Figure 3. (A) Intraoperative endoscopic photographs of the stenotic aqueduct of Sylvius covered with a membrane. (B, C) Fenestration of the membrane and (D) widening of the opening with the aid of the inflation of the balloon catheter. (E) A satisfactory opening is achieved and (F) a multiperforated ventricular catheter tip is introduced into the fourth ventricular space.

After the aqueductoplasty is performed, a multi-perforated ventricular catheter is inserted from the frontal horn of the lateral ventricle via the foramen of Monroe into the third ventricle and through the aqueduct into the fourth ventricle (Figure 3). The catheter is subcutaneously connected to a shunt pump. To avoid any damage to the posterior fossa structures, the length of the catheters should be planned prior to treatment with the help of neuroradiological studies (Figure 4 and 5).

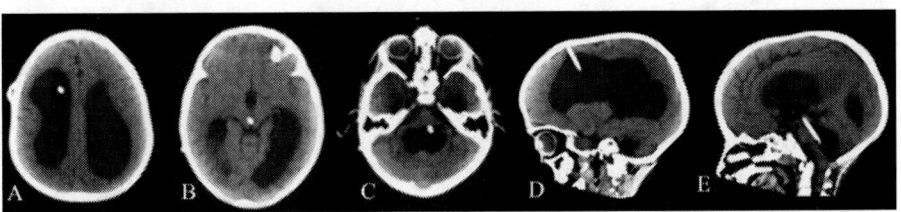

Figure 4. (A, B & C) Axial CT demonstrating the catheter placement at the (A) frontal horn of the right lateral ventricle passing the third ventricle into the (B) Aqueduct of Sylvius and through the aqueduct into the (C) fourth ventricle. (D) Sagittal CT showing the catheter at the frontal horn of the lateral ventricle and (E) catheter tip ending in the fourth ventricle.

The second group according to our algorithm consists of patients where the lateral ventricle and third ventricles are collapsed or small because of a functioning shunt. We further subclassify this group to a type 2(a) and type 2(b). In type 2(a), it is where there is dysmorphism or abnormal shape of the third ventricle, making it anatomically unsuitable for an endoscopic procedure through posterior fossa. In these patients we have practiced externalizing their preexisting shunts to deliberately increase the size of the ventricles until they are deemed favorable for an lateral ventricle endoscopic entry (Figure 6). To follow up and identify the suitable ventricular dilatation needed with no unwanted clinical deterioration of the patient, we perform daily computer tomography (CT) scans of the brain. When this is achieved, we can attempt to proceed with aqueductoplasty via the same supratentorial route as the type 1 patients. This might be one of the setbacks of such an approach as there must be 24-hour availability of a CT scan in a hospital, especially when there is any clinical deterioration during this observation and for daily assessment of the ventricular size.

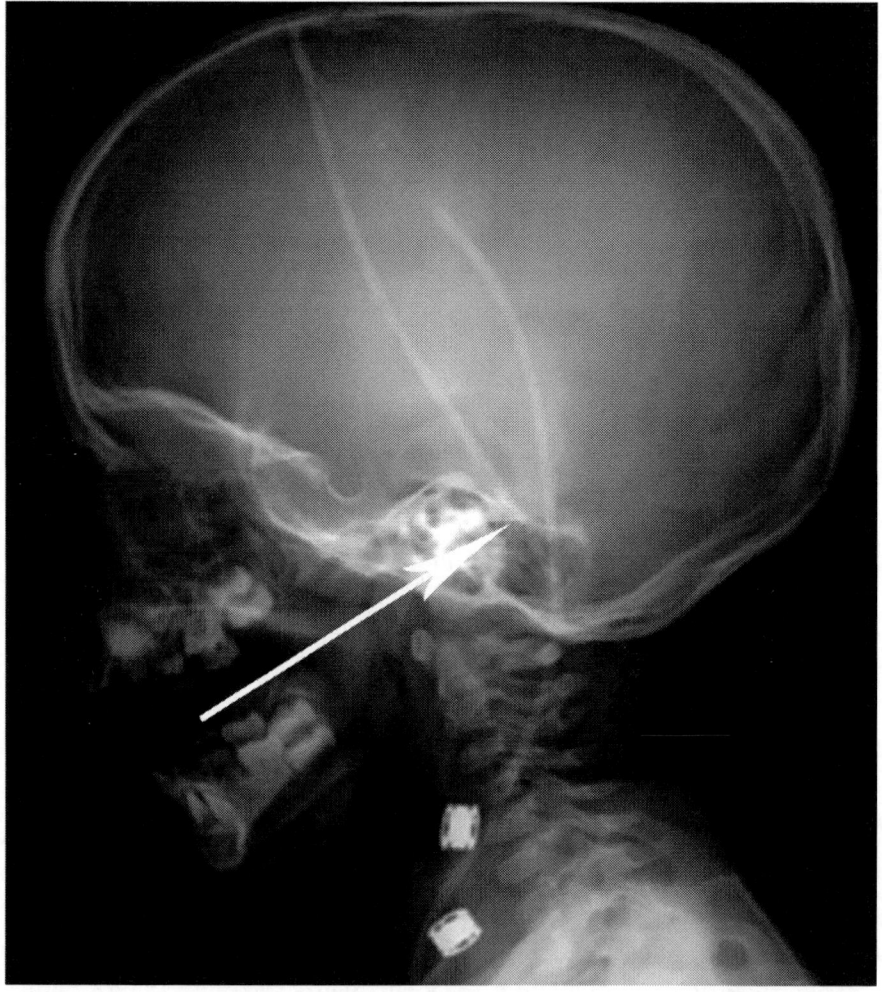

Figure 5. Lateral skull Xray (white arrow) showing the tip of the proximal catheter is in the fourth ventricle.

In type 2(b) the endoscopic route is from below via infratentorial suboccipital approach to the inlet of the fourth ventricle. In these selections of cases, the third ventricular anatomy is normal. There are certain exclusion criteria that need to be identified for a successful outcome with fewer complications. Structural issues such as small third ventricular size and the presence of a large massa intermedia would deem this approach cumbersome and unsuccessful. Moreover, the importance of the trajectory of the endoscope due to anatomical variations – despite the aid of neuronavigation – must be taken into consideration to avoid any unnecessary complication of damage to other nearby neuronal structures.

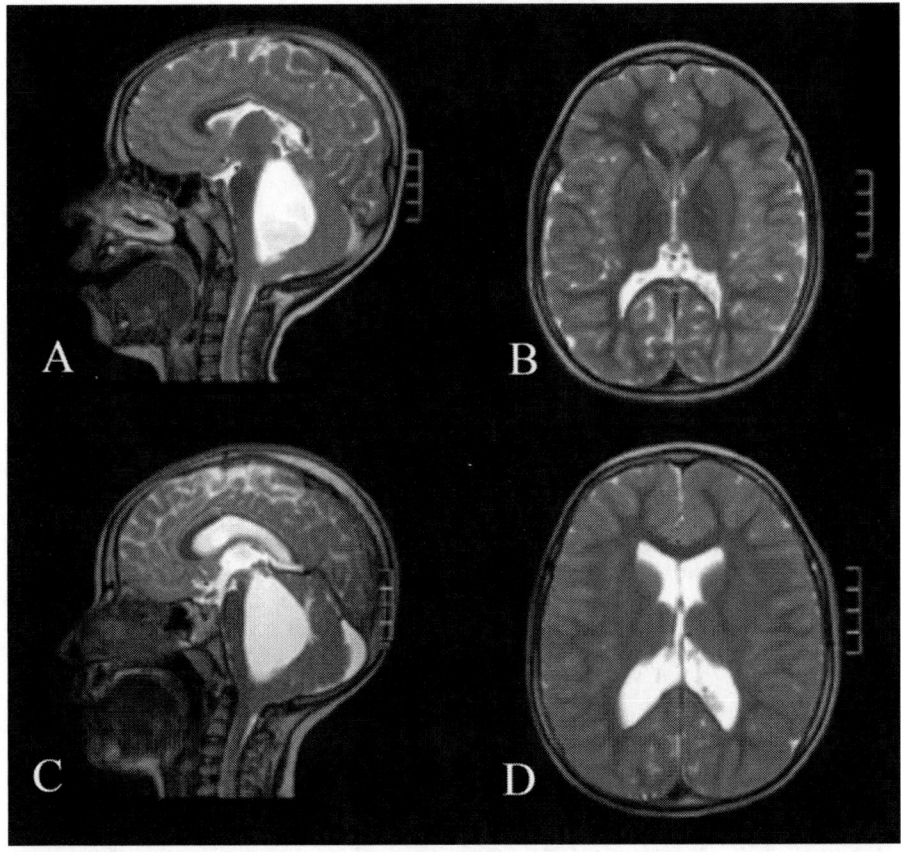

Figure 6. (A) Sagittal T2 MRI showing a huge dilated fourth ventricle and a small decompressed third and lateral ventricle. (B) Axial T2 MRI also demonstrating a slit like appearance of the third and lateral ventricles. (C) Sagittal T2 MRI post externalization of pre-existing shunt revealing a more dilated lateral ventricle for feasibility of endoscopic procedure through it.

For this procedure, the patient is placed in a prone position. The burrhole is made a few centimeters below the transverse sinus and 1 cm lateral to the midline, and with neuronavigation the ideal trajectory is straight and always planned using a 0-degree rigid endoscope with respect to the fourth ventricle [19, 20]. A catheter is introduced from the fourth ventricle towards the aqueduct. Any veil or membranes overlying the inlet are fenestrated initially with a balloon catheter before introducing the ventricular catheter. The catheter is advanced into the third ventricle and subcutaneously connected to an Ommaya reservoir (Figure 7). A control radiological study immediately after surgery is mandatory Figure 8).

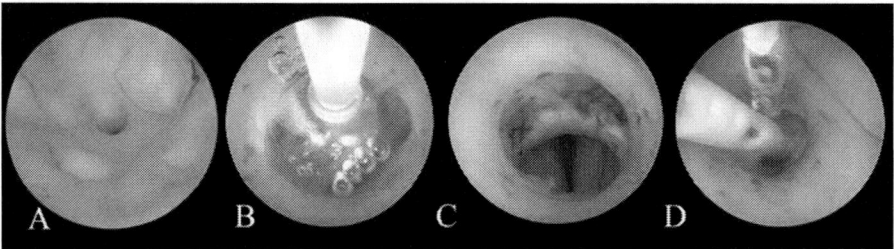

Figure 7. Intraoperative endoscopic photographs demonstrating (A) The stenotic Aqueduct of Sylvius. (B) The aqueduct is fenestrated and dilated with a balloon catheter. (C) After the connection created between the fourth ventricle with dilatation, the roof of the third ventricle is clearly appreciated. (D) A multiperforated catheter is inserted from the fourth ventricle, through the aqueduct into the third ventricle with the help of the double balloon catheter as a guide to the aqueduct.

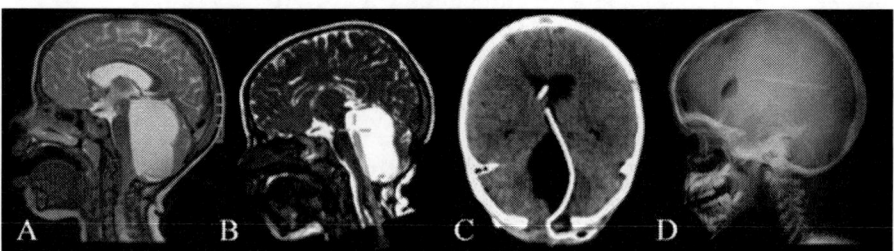

Figure 8. (A) Preoperative sagittal T2 MRI showing a large fourth ventricle. (B) Neuronavigation was used intraoperatively to provide the best trajectory. (C) Postoperative coronal CT showing final placement of the catheter that is connected to an Ommaya reservoir and (D) the preexisting proximal shunt catheter and the additional catheter with Ommaya reservoir demonstrated by this postoperative skull X-ray.

OPEN SURGICAL PROCEDURES

Microsurgical approaches in IFV are not commonly the immediate or first surgical line of treatment mentioned or described. However, this is prudent in cases when endoscopy is not amenable or reserved after all other approaches have failed to provide a favorable outcome.

Villacencio et al., [28] describes suboccipital craniectomy and fenestration of the cyst or entrapped aqueduct and the membranous obstruction of foramen Magendie and Luschka. Arachnoid adhesiolysis was performed in their cases with thickened arachnoid communicating the cyst with spinal subarachnoid space. A similar communicating arachnoidal adhesiolysis was later reported by Udayakumaran et al., [27] where a craniotomy was advocated instead of a craniectomy. In addition to the fenestrations of the fourth ventricular outlet and the veil covered foramen of Magendie, in patients with severe adhesions secondary to arachnoiditis a stent was inserted into the fourth ventricle communicating to the spinal subarachnoid space and anchored to the arachnoid with nonabsorbable sutures.

CONCLUSION

IFV is a challenging pathology to manage. More studies are required to define its pathophysiology and spectrum of surgical treatment available. There is a need to tailor the management accordingly to the carefully selected cases based on the clinico-radiological presentation.

The availability of neuronavigation and neuroendoscopy has widened the scope of management with less morbidity. Developing an algorithm to have a systemic approach with considerations and correlating the radiological factors to the different suitable endoscopic approaches has made selection of the patients with the best outcome possible.

Conflict of Interest

Dr. Jacintha V. Francis attends a pediatric neurosurgery fellowship program in our department which is sponsored by KARL STORZ Company.

References

[1] Ang B. T., Steinbok P., Cochrane D. D. 2006. "Etiological differences between the isolated lateral ventricle and isolated fourth ventricle." *Childs Nerv. Syst.* Sep; 22(9): 1080-5.
[2] Barami, K., Chakrabarti, I., Silverthorn, J., Ciporen, J., & Akins, P. T. 2018." Diagnosis, Classification, and Management of Fourth Ventriculomegaly in Adults: Report of 9 Cases and Literature Review." *World Neurosurgery*, 116, e709–e722.
[3] Cinnali G., Spennato P., Savarese L., et al., 2006. "Endoscopic aqueductoplasty and placement of a stent in the cerebral aqueduct in the management of isolated fourth ventricle in children." *J. Neurosurgery* 104:21-27.
[4] Coker, S. B. 1986. "Bobble-head doll syndrome due to trapped fourth ventricle and aqueduct." *Pediatric Neurology*, 2(2), 115–116.
[5] Folts E. L., De Feo Dr. 1980." Double compartment hydrocephalus – a new clinical entity." *Neurosurgery* 7:551-559.
[6] Fritsch, M. J., Lienke, S., Manwaring, K. H., & Mehdorn, H. M. 2004. "Endoscopic Aqueductoplasty and Interventriculostomy for the treatment of Isolated Fourth Ventricle in Children." *Neurosurgery*, 55(2), 372-379.
[7] Gallo, P., Hermier, M., Mottolese, C., Ricci-Franchi, A.-C., Rousselle, C., Simon, E., & Szathmari, A. 2012. "The endoscopic trans-fourth ventricle aqueductoplasty and stent placement for the treatment of trapped fourth ventricle: Long-term results in a series of 18 consecutive patients." *Neurology India*, 60(3), 271.

[8] Harter D. H. 2004. "Management strategies for treatment of trapped fourth ventricle." *Childs Nerv. syst.* 20:710-716.

[9] Hawkin J. C. III, Hoffman H. J., Humphreys R. P. 1978. "Isolated fourth ventricle as a complication of ventricular shunting. Report of three cases." *J. Neurosurg.* 49: 910-913.

[10] James H. E. 1990-91. "Spectrum of the syndrome of the isolated fourth ventricle in post hemorrhagic hydrocephalus of premature infants." *Pediatr. Neurosurg.* 16: 305-308.

[11] Little, A. S., Zabramski, J. M., & Nakaji, P. N. 2010. "Simplified Aqueductal Stenting for Isolated Fourth Ventricle Using a Small-Caliber Flexible Endoscope in a Patient with Neurococcidiomycosis." *Operative Neurosurgery*, 66, onsE373–onsE374.

[12] Lunsfard, L. D. 2007. "Trapped IV ventricle." *Journal of Neurosurgery: Pediatrics*, 106(4), 330-330.

[13] Mohanty, A., & Manwaring, K. 2017. "Isolated Fourth Ventricle: To Shunt or Stent." *Operative Neurosurgery*, 14(5), 483–493.

[14] Montes J. L., Clarke D. B., Farmer J. P. 1994. "Stereotactic transtentorial hiatus ventriculoperitoneal shunting for the sequestrated fourth ventricle. Technical note." *J. Neurosurg.* 80:759-761.

[15] Montgomery, C. T., & Winfield, J. A. 1993. "Fourth Ventricular Entrapment Caused by Rostrocaudal Herniation following Shunt Malfunction." *Pediatric Neurosurgery*, 19(4), 209–214.

[16] Parker Mickle, J., & Friedman, W. A. 1981." Encysted fourth ventricle." *Surgical Neurology*, 16(2), 150-153.

[17] Raimondi, A. J., Samuelson, G., Yarzagaray, L., & Norton, T. 1969. "Atresia of the Foramina of Luschka and Magendie: The Dandy-Walker Cyst." *Journal of Neurosurgery*, 31(2), 202–216.

[18] Rohde, V., Behm, T., Ludwig, H., & Wachter, D. 2011. "The role of neuronavigation in intracranial endoscopic procedures." *Neurosurgical Review*, 35(3), 351–358.
[19] Sansone, J. M., & Iskandar, B. J. 2005. "Endoscopic cerebral aqueductoplasty: a trans-fourth ventricle approach." *Journal of Neurosurgery: Pediatrics*, 103(5), 388–392.
[20] Say, I., Dodson, V., Tomycz, L., & Mazzola, C. 2019. "Endoscopic Fourth Ventriculostomy: Suboccipital Transaqueductal Approach for Fenestration of an Isolated Fourth Ventricle, Case Report and Technical Note." *World Neurosurgery*.
[21] Scotti, G., Musgrave, M., Fitz, C., & Harwood-Nash, D. 1980. "The isolated fourth ventricle in children: CT and clinical review of 16 cases." *American Journal of Roentgenology*, 135(6), 1233–123.
[22] Sharma R. R., Pawar S. J., Devadas R. V., Dev E. J. 2001. "CT stereotaxy guided lateral transcerebellar programmable fourth ventriculo- peritoneal shunting for symptomatic trapped fourth ventricle." *Clin. Neurol. Neurosurg.* 103: 143-146.
[23] Shin M., Morita A., Asano S., Ueki K., Kirino T. 2000. "Neuroendoscopic aqueductal stent placement for isolated fourth ventricle. Case report." *J. Neurosurg.* 92: 1036-1039.
[24] Shose Y., Nagaki H., Kamikawa S. 1991. "Disproportionately large communicating fourth ventricle. Case report." *Neurol. Med. Chir.* (Tokyo) 31: 1003-1007.
[25] Teo, C., Kadrian, D., & Hayhurst, C. 2013. "Endoscopic Management of Complex Hydrocephalus." *World Neurosurgery*, 79(2), S21.e1–S21.e7.
[26] Udayakumaran, S., Bo, X., Ben Sira, L., & Constantini, S. 2009. "Unusual subacute diencephalic edema associated with a trapped fourth ventricle: resolution following foramen magnum decompression." *Child's Nervous System*, 25(11), 1517–1520.

[27] Udayakumaran, S., Biyani, N., Rosenbaum, D. P., Ben-Sira, L., Constantini, S., & Beni-Adani, L. 2011. "Posterior fossa craniotomy for trapped fourth ventricle in shunt-treated hydrocephalic children: long-term outcome." *Journal of Neurosurgery: Pediatrics*, 7(1), 52–63.
[28] Villavicencio, A. T., Wellons III, J. C., & George, T. M. 1998. "Avoiding Complicated Shunt Systems by Open Fenestration of Symptomatic Fourth Ventricular Cysts Associated with Hydrocephalus." *Pediatric Neurosurgery*, 29(6), 314–319.

In: Neuroendoscopic Procedures ...
Editor: Soner Duru
ISBN: 978-1-68507-092-2
© 2021 Nova Science Publishers, Inc.

Chapter 3

RADIOLOGICAL EVALUATION OF THE STOMA PATENCY IN INTRAVENTRICULAR FENESTRATIONS

Aydan Arslan[1], Alp Dincer[2] and M. Memet Özek[3]

[1]Instructor of Radiology,
Zonguldak Maternity and Child Health Hospital, Turkey
[2]Professor of Radiology, Department of Radiology,
Acıbadem University, School of Medicine, Istanbul – Turkey
[3]Professor of Neurosurgery, Head, Department of Neurosurgery,
Chief, Division of Pediatric Neurosurgery,
Acıbadem University, School of Medicine, Istanbul – Turkey

ABSTRACT

Intraventricular endoscopic fenestration is a popular alternative treatment method that has been increasingly used in recent years. Radiological imaging tools are very important to manage these cases during preoperative, postoperative and follow-up period. In preoperative evaluation, imaging aims to show hydrocephalus status, appropriateness of endoscopic treatment and other pathologies. Postoperative and follow-up imaging will assess the efficacy of the endoscopic fenestration, state of hydrocephalus, cyst size, and possible complications.

Keywords: hydrocephalus, radiologic assessment, intraventricular fenestrations, 3D SPACE T2, 3D CISS, MRI, endoscopic third ventriculostomy, cyst ventriculostomy, fourth ventriculostomy, septum pellucidum fenestration

INTRODUCTION

Intraventricular endoscopic fenestrations are simple, minimally invasive well-accepted treatment modalities. In recent years, different types of fenestrations have been frequently used to reduce mortality and morbidity due to shunting or open surgery. Nowoslawska E. et al. (2003) reported that neuroendoscopic techniques have better clinical results and fewer complications compared to shunt implantation in patients with complicated hydrocephalus. Endoscopic procedures would provide patients with an opportunity to be shunt independent.

Appropriate endoscopic treatment is planned according to the underlying reason for hydrocephalus in pediatric cases. Endoscopic third ventriculostomy, septostomy, foraminoplasty, cystoventriculostomy, fourth ventriculostomy are some of the methods defined as intraventricular fenestration in the literature. Radiological evaluation plays a crucial role in pre-operative treatment planning and post-operative patient follow-up and management.

Computed tomography cisternography (CTC), Magnetic resonance (MR) cisternography, phase-contrast (PC) Cine MR, 3D CISS (three-dimensional constructive interference in steady state), and 3D SPACE T2 sequences, in addition to routine brain MRI sequences, have been used in the evaluation of stoma flow from past to present (Dinçer A., Özek MM, 2011).

PATENCY ASSESSMENT OF ENDOSCOPIC THIRD VENTRICULOSTOMY

Endoscopic third ventriculostomy (ETV) is a minimally invasive surgical method that provides communication between the third ventricle and the interpeduncular cistern with a permanent defect on the floor of the third ventricle in obstructive hydrocephalus patients. Aqueductal stenosis, posterior fossa tumors, shunt malfunction, Dandy-Walker malformation, and Blake's pouch are some of the indications of ETV (Dinçer A. et al. 2011).

Aqueductal stenosis (AS) is the most frequent indication of ETV and the most common cause of congenital obstructive hydrocephalus. Symptoms and/or signs develop secondary to hydrocephalus and increased intracranial pressure. AS is frequently seen congenitally in children and acquired in adults. It can be idiopathic or secondary to a known etiology. Congenital causes include aqueductal webs or diaphragms. Tumor-related compression, vascular malformations, hemorrhage, and infections are some of the acquired causes (Little JR. et al. 1975; El Damaty A. et al. 2020).

Characteristic antenatal ultrasound findings of aqueductal stenosis are triventricular dilation; enlargement of both lateral and third ventricles. Posterior fossa details and investigation for the aqueduct, the floor of the third ventricle, and the foramen magnum may not be seen very clearly, dependent on the fontanel opening. Other causes of hydrocephalus may not be reliably excluded (Dinçer A. et al. 2011).

Preoperative and postoperative evaluation plays an essential role in the prevention of possible complications and follow-up in patients with ETV. The anatomy of the lateral ventricles and the third ventricle, foramen Monroe width, presence of obstructive membrane, position of the basilar artery, presence of severe skull base anomaly should be detected in preoperative evaluation. In the postoperative period, with conventional MR sequences, midsagittal surgical defect of the floor of the third ventricle, resolution of periventricular edema, widening of subarachnoid space, regression of hydrocephalus, possible post-operative complications are detected (Dinçer A. et al. 2011). Conventional MR sequences for this protocol are sagittal-axial-coronal T2, axial T1, sagittal 3D T2 flair, diffusion, and axial 3D SWI. Conventional MR sequences are inadequate to show flow patterns due to poor spatial resolution and flow effect. In addition to conventional sequences, evaluation should include detailed 3D CISS sequence (Dinçer A. et al. 2011).

CTC and MRC are used for ETV stoma patency evaluation; however, due to intrathecal interventions, non-invasive techniques have been replaced by long-term follow-up of these patients worldwide. Cine PC is a qualitative and quantitative technique in evaluating flow through the ETV fenestration. However, the disadvantages are that the complex CCF flow does not show sufficient efficacy, may under or overestimate flow, and show false-positive results (Yildiz H. et al. 2005). It also needs to be evaluated simultaneously by an experienced neuroradiologist. Morphological data cannot be given with the PC CINE sequence. Quantitative evaluation can be done with PC CINE, but no cutoff value was found in daily routine practice. (Algin O. et al. 2015).

Schwartz TH. et al. (1996) demonstrated that in the postoperative period (one month), third ventricular width was a more reliable indicator in determining prognosis. A decrease in the third ventricular width by at least 15% was seen in all successful cases and none of the failures. Changes in ventricular size alone did not fully predict surgical outcome. In some cases of ETV, closed stoma and dysfunction, a decrease in ventricle size can be seen. Evaluation of stoma patency is one of the most objective indicators in determining surgical success or failure (Kim SK. et al. 2000).

Functional ETV stoma confirms with the demonstration of signal void using sagittal T2 3D SPACE sequence. No advantages of PC-MRI and 3D heavily T2W techniques over the 3D-SPACE technique could be shown in the assessment of ETV patency (Algin O. et al. 2015). The presence of newly developed thin membrane and adhesion are questioned with the 3D CISS sequence (Dinçer A. et al. 2011). When used in combination, 3D-SPACE T2 and 3D CISS sequence can provide reliable information of the anatomy of the CSF pathways, the site of obstruction, potential operative targets for intervention, and the functionality of the stoma.

A study involving 29 cases showed VFD (third ventricle floor depression), LTB (lamina terminalis bowing), ACTC (Anterior commissure − tuber cinereum distance), MBLT (mamillary body−lamina terminalis distance), and TVW (third ventricular width) were significantly reduced in successful ETV patients. There was no association with lateral ventricular measurements (Börcek AÖ. et al. 2017). Evaluation of treatment success is based on radiological evaluation and improvement of symptoms before surgery.

Kombogiorgas D et al. (2006) reported that the success rate of ETV depends on stoma size, CSF leak was strongly associated with failure. Other factors such as the presence of pre-pontine adhesions, thick or double floor of the third ventricle did not prove association with ETV success.

A series of 29 hydrocephalic children with ETV in whom postoperative sagittal T1-weighted and T2-weighted images of flow void were present in 94% of successes and absent in 75% of failures, this was statistically significant ($p = 0.01$). There were no significant differences between the mean ventricular reductions in both groups (Kulkarni AV. et al. 2000). Lucic MA. Et al. (2014) demonstrated the absence of a reduction in ventricle volume in almost one-third of the patients with both clinical and dynamic MRI signs of successful ETV in the early postoperative period. An early postoperative MRI is overly sensitive to failure of ETV, but not highly specific (Udayakumaran S. et al. 2019).

PATENCY ASSESSMENT OF SEPTUM PELLUCIDUM FENESTRATION

Septum pellucidum is a 1.5-3.0 mm thin, single membrane located in the brain between the body and anterior horns of the lateral ventricles. Extending from the corpus callosum to the fornix consisting of two fused leaves. The function of the septum pellucidum is not well known (Sarwar M. 1989). A narrow cavity (or a potential cavity) between the two leaves can be seen; this structure is named persistent CSP (cavum septum pellucidum) rostrally and persistent cavum vergae caudally. If the cavum septum pellucidum leaves are damaged, free CSF flow occurs between the lateral ventricles (Griffiths PD. et al. 2009). The septum pellucidum develops at 10-12 weeks of gestation from the primitive lamina terminalis or the commissural plate and is fully developed by 17 weeks of gestation (Sarwar M. 1989). It is closely related to the development of the corpus callosum and fornix (Rakic P. et al. 1968).

There are approximately two septal veins in the septum pellucidum and no arteries. The anterior area of septum pellucidum is consistently avascular and large enough to be fenestrated safely. More posterior areas, while avascular, are not suitable in size and shape (Vinas FC. et al. 1998). Notably recommended for intervention is the anterior area of the middle septal region, at the level of the foramen of Monroe, mid-height between the corpus callosum and fornix (Roth J. et al. 2010).

Septum pellucidum fenestration (septostomy) indication is all lesions that obstruct foramen Monroe. Septum pellucidum cysts; multiloculated cystic hydrocephalus; neoplastic processes; membranous obstruction; inflammatory isolated lateral ventricle; giant aneurysm; congenital atresia; and vascular malformations are some of the indications of septostomy described in the literature (Oertel JM et al. 2009, Tubbs RS. et al. 2014).

Preoperative radiological evaluation is essential in patients with septum pellucidum fenestration to avoid injury to a contralateral large septal vein (Roth J. et al. 2010). According to our experience, thin slice, fat-sat post-contrast T1-weighted sequence, and SWI sequence can be used to evaluate septal veins. Besides, MRI is necessary to determine the etiology of foramen Monroe obstruction. With conventional MR sequences, cavum septum pellucidum dilated lateral ventricles, and normal sized third ventricle is observed. With the 3D CISS sequence, obstruction of the foramen Monroe, possible thin membranes, and adhesions are easily visualized. No flow through the foramina of Monroe is observed with the 3D SPACE T2 sequence.

Postoperative radiological evaluation plays a key role in the evaluation of surgical success and follow-up as in other neuroendoscopic procedures.

Conventional MR sequences show resolution of the hydrocephalus, endoscopic fenestration of the septum pellucidum, and possible post-op complications. The combination of the 3D CISS sequence and 3D SPACE T2 sequences gives detailed information about the anatomy and flow pattern of the endoscopic stoma.

PATENCY ASSESSMENT OF AQUEDUCTOPLASTY

Endoscopic aqueductoplasty (EA) is an effective alternative to the third ventriculostomy for the treatment of hydrocephalus caused by membranous and/or short-segment stenosis of the aqueduct (da Silva LRF. et al. 2007). Neuroendoscopic aqueductoplasty allows free communication between the fourth ventricle and the supratentorial ventricular system.

The advantages of EA compared to ETV are, an increased physiological cerebrospinal fluid (CSF) pathway without risk of basilar artery injury, damage to the hypothalamus and less traumatic access to arachnoid adhesions (Schroeder HW. et al. 2004, Schroeder HW, et al. 1999).

Aqueductoplasty is riskier than the third ventriculostomy because of surrounding delicate midbrain structures. However, with advanced endoscopic techniques and surgeon experience, EA can be performed safely in carefully selected patients. Reopening the aqueduct in long stenoses carries a high risk of midbrain injury with neurological problems, such as disconjugate eye movement, Parinaud's syndrome, and oculomotor or trochlear palsy. ETV is the best treatment method in this patient group. The size of the aqueductal stenosis is important in planning treatment, while EA is recommended in short stenosis (less than 5 mm in size) and ETV is recommended in long stenosis (Schroeder HW, et al. 1999). These endoscopic treatments can be applied alone or in combination according to the patient's status.

Proper patient selection is important in this endoscopic procedure and is planned with preoperative MRI imaging. By means of conventional MR sequences, triventricular hydrocephalus, bulging of the floor of the third ventricle, aqueductal obstruction or aqueductal stenosis and edema surrounding the lateral ventricles can be easily visualized. Conventional MR sequences are insufficient in showing very thin intra-aqueductal membranes and arachnoid membranes within the prepontine cisterns and CSF flow within the aqueduct. These can be best seen in the combination of the 3D CISS sequence and 3D SPACE T2 sequences.

Lifelong follow-up examinations are mandatory for all endoscopically treated patients. Postoperatively, conventional MR sequences show resolution of the hydrocephalus, endoscopic ventriculostomy site, and possible post-operative complications.

PATENCY ASSESSMENT OF CYSTOVENTRICULOSTOMY STOMAS

Arachnoid cysts are benign, well-defined lesions containing cerebrospinal fluid (CSF). In a consecutive series of adult patients undergoing intracranial imaging; the prevalence of 1.4% was found (Al-Holou, WN et al. 2013) The prevalence of arachnoid cysts recorded was 2.6% in a large population of children; higher than prior estimates in adults (Al-Holou, WN et al. 2010).

The best diagnostic clues for identifying arachnoid cysts are cysts with smooth contour extra-axial CSF density. Scalloping due to compression can be seen in the adjacent bone structure. (Osborn AG et al. 2006). Epidermoid cyst is frequently found in the differential diagnosis. No diffusion restriction, suppression in the Flair sequence identical to CSF, usually uniocular and displace adjacent arteries and cranial nerves rather than engulf them are the features that distinguish the arachnoid cyst from the epidermoid cyst (Osborn AG et al. 2006). Subdural hygroma (chronic subdural hemorrhage) is another differential diagnosis. Subdural hygroma does not have CSF signal intensity on MR images and often has an enhancing membrane. Porencephalic cysts, usually surrounded by gliosis, have a history of trauma or stroke. Cystic neoplasms can also be confused for arachnoid cysts. It can be distinguished from cystic neoplasm because it does not contain solid or contrasting components and it is extra-axial (Osborn AG 2004).

Arachnoid cysts are generally asymptomatic. It was observed that approximately 5% of cases are symptomatic. Arachnoid cysts located at the sellar/suprasellar, ambient cistern, quadrigeminal, and cerebellopontine angle were observed to be more symptomatic. It was observed to be symptomatic due to an increase in cyst size and consequent mass effect leading to hydrocephalus and neurological symptoms (Al-Holou, WN et al. 2013).

Most arachnoid cysts do not require treatment. Patients requiring treatment who are symptomatic and those with increased cyst size during follow-up (Arslan A et al. 2019). There are a lot of treatment options of arachnoid cysts published up to date such as open craniotomy for cyst excision, neuroendoscopic fenestration, microsurgical fenestration, or cystoperitoneal shunt (Ali ZS. et al. 2014). On the other hand, there is no ideal method. The treatment selected depends on the personal experience of the surgeon and radiological features of the cyst (Rodriguez JF. et al. 2014).

Each method offers unique advantages and disadvantages. Cystoventriculostomy and cystosternostomy are effective treatment modalities due to rapid recovery time, less morbidity and mortality, low rate of repetitive surgical procedures, and persistent worsening (Nowosławska E. et al. 2006), avoiding shunt-induced infection and other complications (Rodriguez JF. et al. 2014). Neuroendoscopy is a microinvasive procedure closest to physiology (Özek MM. et al. 2013) (Arslan A et al. 2019).

Radiological evaluation plays an objective diagnostic role in the follow-up of cases treated with the neuro endoscopy method. Clinical symptoms and physical examination can be misleading, especially in pediatric patients.

Computed tomography cisternography (CTC) is an imaging technique, could provide a real-time evaluation of CSF movement. The non-ionic low-osmolar contrast agent is given to the thecal sac after lumbar puncture.

Post-contrast images are then compared with the pre-contrast image; preoperative communicating and non-communicating arachnoid cyst differential diagnosis can be made based on contrast filling time (Wang X et al. 2012). Stoma patency can be evaluated by computed tomography cisternography, but it is one of the disadvantages that it contains ionized radiation, the use of contrast agent (due to contrast agent allergy), and is an invasive method.

Magnetic resonance cisternography (MRC) a heavily T2-weighted fast spin-echo sequence that enhances the signal intensity of the cerebrospinal fluid (CSF) with subtraction of the background (El Gammal T. et al. 1994). MR contrast agent is also given from intrathecal space at the lower lumbar region. According to intracystic contrast agent involvement, communications between the arachnoid cysts and the CSF pathways of the CNS are considered. MRC does not contain ionized radiation and bony artifact also it can take multiplanar images (Tali ET. et al. 2004). Despite the advantages of MRC, it is among the disadvantages of being invasive, risk of complications secondary to intrathecal intervention, risk of gadolinium-based contrast agent allergy, and suspicious findings in intraventricular cysts (Algın O. et al. 2009).

Phase-contrast (PC) Cine MR imaging is a noninvasive MRI technique-based phase shift between flowing and stationary nuclei to be used to visualize CSF movement. CSF circulation is pulsatile, synchronous with the cardiac rhythm. Cardiac-gated MRI using phase contrast is more sensitive (Connor SEJ et al. 2001). PC MRI may improve the diagnostic confidence in differentiating between communicating and non-communicating arachnoid cyst (Battal B. et al. 2011). Jet flow (black or white flow) in the arachnoid cyst to be a reliable finding showing communicating arachnoid cyst (Eguchi T. et al. 1996). The qualitative flow data can obtain with a 2D fast low-angle shot (FLASH) gradient-echo sequence, gradient- recalled acquisition in the steady-state [GRASS], or PSIF sequence (Steady-State Free Precession (SSFP) imaging technique) (Yildiz H. et al. 2005). It does not contain ionizing radiation; no contrast agent is required. The acquisition time of PC-MRI was approximately 5 min depends on the patient's heart rate (Algın O. et al. 2009). PC sequences are more suitable for evaluating laminar flow. Therefore, its sensitivity may decrease in evaluation low turbulent and complex CCF flow and false-positive results can be obtained (Yildiz H. et al. 2005). PC Cine MR shows only CSF flow, it is unable to demonstrate cisternal anatomic details. PC Cine MR demonstrates only bidirectional flow in a selected direction. Images can be taken from different regions, but the time will be longer. Aliasing artifacts can be seen, radiologist experience is important in prevention (Dinçer A. et al. 2011).

Conventional MR sequences show arachnoid cyst size (preoperative-postoperative changes), hydrocephalus, midline shift, compression findings on other structures, brain parenchyma findings, possible complications (bleeding ... etc.) in patients undergoing cystoventriculostomy (Arslan A et al. 2019). In neuroendoscopic procedures, demonstrating the level of obstruction and stoma patency is a key issue. Conventional MR sequences give us limited information on this, due to poor spatial resolution, the poor contrast-to-noise ratio between the cisterns and neighboring structures, and CSF flow effects (Dinçer A. et al. 2009).

Three-dimensional constructive interference in the steady-state (synonyms (DRIVE-BFE (Philips), CISS (Siemens), FIESTA (GE)) and 3D SPACE T2 sequences play a crucial role in the assessment of CSF flow dynamics as well as a better understanding of cystoventriculostomy stoma patency. 3D CISS is a flow-compensated gradient-echo sequence that gives not only anatomical details on fine membranous obstructive structures within the ventricles, aqueduct, cisterns, and CSF pathway but also improved the orientation of the surgeon. The image contrast of the CISS sequence determines the T2/T1 ratio of the tissue (Chavhan GB. et al. 2008). A high signal is obtained from tissues that have long T2 relaxation times and short T1 relaxation times such as CCF (Hingwala D. et al. 2011). 3D CISS imaging provides excellent spatial resolution and CSF/brain tissue contrast, compared with conventional T2-weighted sequences (Aleman J. et al. 2001). The desired region can be evaluated in detail with multiplanar reconstruction technique (Yang D. Et al. 2000) thin membranes.

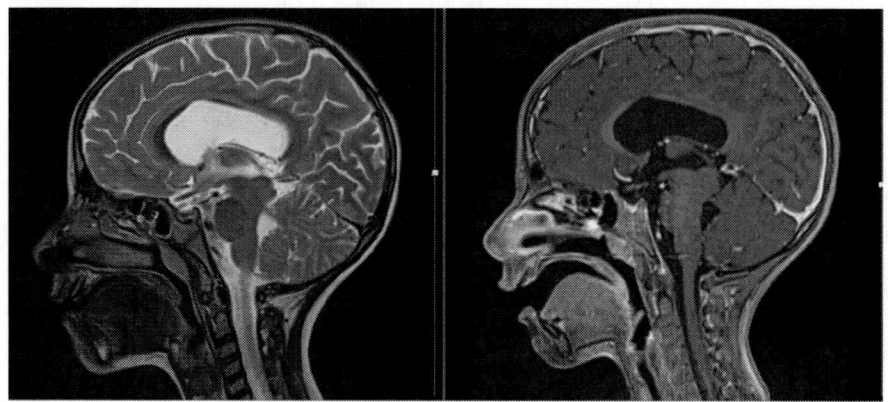

Figure 1. The TSE T2 sagittal and post contrast T1 images of an 8 years-old girl with a tectal plate glioma demonstrates the persisting ventriculomegaly. The stoma defect at the tuber cinerium level is obvious.

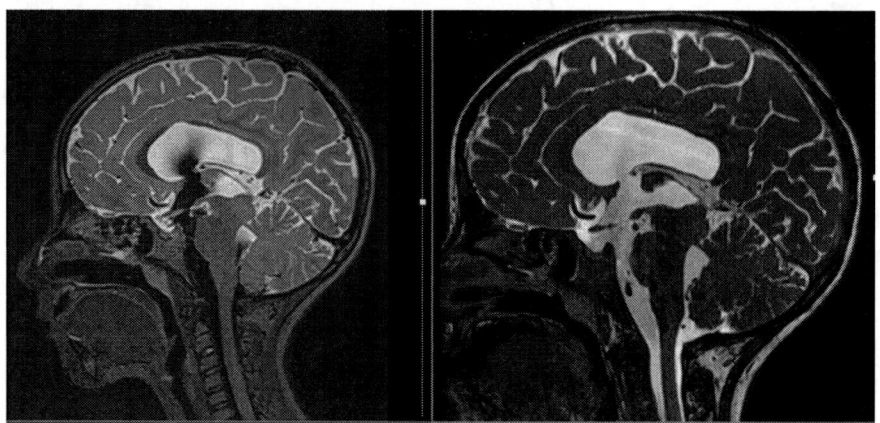

Figure 2. The 3D CISS and 3D SPACE T2 sequences of the same case show that the ETV stoma is anatomically open and functional.

Since the 3D CISS sequence is a GRE sequence, aliasing and susceptibility artifacts can be seen; lowering the flip angle and increasing the receiver bandwidth can help eliminate these artifacts. It has poor tissue contrast, so brain parenchymal imaging sensitivity is low; gray-white matter differentiation is also not well visualized (Dinçer A. et al. 2011). Acquisition time is approximately 4.32min; due to the relatively long time, motion artifacts could be problematic; sedation can be a problem solver in these cases especially under the age of ten. Banding artifacts are rarely seen, but the real-artifacts distinction can be made easily due to its specific shape (Dinçer A. et al. 2009). One of the limitations of the 3D CISS sequence; it is not useful in the assessment of flow through the fenestration (Dinçer A. et al. 2011).

3D SPACE T2 (sampling perfection with application-optimized contrasts using different flip angle evolution) uses different flip angles, can be obtained thin-sectioned images with a good spatial resolution (JPIII M. Et al. 2001). 3D SPACE sequence provides a noninvasive evaluation of CSF flow like PC-MRI. In the part where CSF without obstruction moves freely, the hypointense signal is observed Average acquisition time is 4.21min; It can provide sufficient physiological and morphological data alone with multiplanar reformatted images with high resolution (Algin O. et al. 2012). 3D SPACE T2 sequence has no flow compensation (gradient-moment nulling); it also minimizes partial volume effect (Arslan A et al. 2019). One of the 3D SPACE T2 limitations does not allow quantitative evaluation (Algin O. et al. 2015).

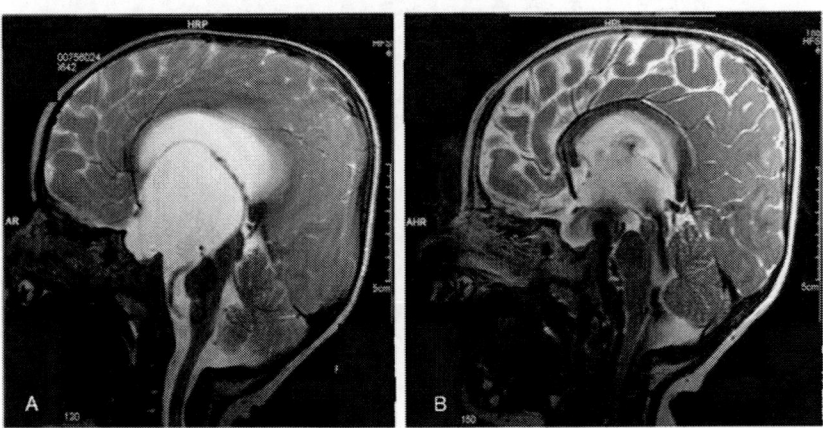

Figure 3. A. A huge suprasellar arachnoid cyst presenting significant displacement of brain stem and no flow through the aqueduct. B. After successful ventriculocystosisternostomy the chiasm and mammillary bodies reoriented to a more normal anatomical position. There is CSF flow through the fenestrations and the aqueduct.

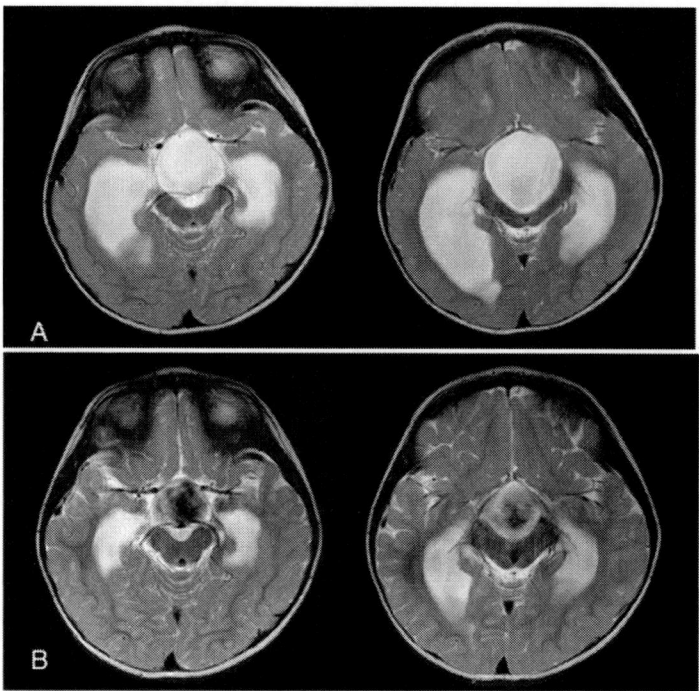

Figure 4. A. Preoperative axial cut of the same case presenting severe hydrocephalus. B. Immediately after surgery the ventricle size diminished and the flow through the fenestrations is satisfactory.

3D SPACE T2 and 3D CISS sequences in addition to conventional sequences are useful in detecting stoma patency and follow-up examinations after cystosternostomy or cystoventriculostomy procedure. MRI findings also correlate with postoperative results in this patient group (Arslan A et al. 2019).

Conclusion

Radiological evaluation plays important role in the preop, postop, and follow-up of patients with neuroendoscopic fenestration.

REFERENCES

Özek, M. M., & Urgun, K. 2013. "Neuroendoscopic management of suprasellar arachnoid cysts." *World neurosurgery* 79(2), S19-e13.

AG., Osborn. 2004. "Arachnoid cyst." *Diagnostic imaging: brain* içinde, yazan A. G., Blaser, S. I., Salzman, K. L., Katzman, G. L., Provenzale, J., & Castillo, M. Osborn, I-7-4. Salt Lake City, Utah: Amirsys.

Aleman, J., Jokura, H., Higano, S., Akabane, A., Shirane, R., Yoshimoto, T. 2001. "Value of constructive interference in steady-state, three-dimensional, Fourier transformation magnetic resonance imaging for the neuroendoscopic treatment of hydrocephalus and intracranial cysts." *Neurosurgery* 48(6), 1291-1296.

Algın, O., Hakyemez, B., Gokalp, G., Korfalı, E., Parlak, M. 2009. "Phase-contrast cine MRI versus MR cisternography on the evaluation of the communication between intraventricular arachnoid cysts and neighbouring cerebrospinal fluid spaces." *Neuroradiology* 51(5), 305-312.

Algin, O., Turkbey, B. 2012. "Evaluation of aqueductal stenosis by 3D sampling perfection with application-optimized contrasts using different flip angle evolutions sequence: preliminary results with 3T MR imaging." *American journal of neuroradiology* 33(4), 740-746.

Algin, O., Ucar, M., Ozmen, E., Borcek, A. O., Ozisik, P., Ocakoglu, G., & Tali, E. T. 2015. "Assessment of third ventriculostomy patency with the 3D-SPACE technique: a preliminary multicenter research study." *Journal of neurosurgery* 122(6), 1347-1355.

Al-Holou, W. N., Terman, S., Kilburg, C., Garton, H. J., Muraszko, K. M., Maher, C. O. 2013. "Prevalence and natural history of arachnoid cysts in adults." *Journal of neurosurgery* 118(2), 222-231.

Al-Holou, W. N., Yew, A. Y., Boomsaad, Z. E., Garton, H. J., Muraszko, K. M., & Maher, C. O. 2010. "Prevalence and natural history of arachnoid cysts in children." *Journal of Neurosurgery: Pediatrics* 5(6), 578-585.

Ali, Z. S., Lang, S. S., Bakar, D., Storm, P. B., Stein, S. C. 2014. "Pediatric intracranial arachnoid cysts: comparative effectiveness of surgical treatment options." *Child's Nervous System* 30(3), 461-469.

Arslan, A., Başarır, M., Özek, M. M., & Dinçer, A. 2019. "Postoperative patency assessment of Cystocisternostomy and Cystoventriculostomy stomas in cases with Arachnoidal cyst." *Child's Nervous System* 1-9.

Börcek, A. Ö., Uçar, M., Karaaslan, B. 2017. "Simplest radiological measurement related to clinical success in endoscopic third ventriculostomy." *Clinical neurology and neurosurgery* 152, 16-22.

Battal, B., Kocaoglu, M., Bulakbasi, N., Husmen, G., Tuba Sanal, H., Tayfun, C. 2011. "Cerebrospinal fluid flow imaging by using phase-contrast MR technique. ." *The British journal of radiology* 84(1004), 758-765.

Chavhan GB, Babyn PS, Jankharia BG, Cheng HL, Shroff MM. 2008. "Steady-State MR Imaging Sequences: Physics, Classification, and Clinical Applications." *Radiographics* 28:1147-60.

Connor, S. E. J., O'Gorman, R., Summers, P., Simmons, A., Moore, E. M., Chandler, C., Jarosz, J. M. 2001. "SPAMM, cine phase contrast imaging and fast spin-echo T2-weighted imaging in the study of intracranial cerebrospinal fluid (CSF) flow." *Clinical radiology* 56(9), 763-772.

da Silva, L. R. F., Cavalheiro, S., Zymberg, S. T. 2007. "Endoscopic aqueductoplasty in the treatment of aqueductal stenosis." *Child's Nervous System* 23(11), 1263-1268.

Dinçer, A., & Özek, M. M. 2011. "Radiologic evaluation of pediatric hydrocephalus." *Child's Nervous System* 27(10), 1543.

Dinçer, A., Kohan, S., Özek, M. M. (2009). "Is all "communicating" hydrocephalus really communicating? Prospective study on the value of 3D-constructive interference in steady state sequence at 3T. ." *American journal of neuroradiology* 30(10), 1898-1906.

Dinçer, A., Yildiz, E., Kohan, S., Özek, M. M. 2011. "Analysis of endoscopic third ventriculostomy patency by MRI: value of different pulse sequences, the sequence parameters, and the imaging planes for investigation of flow void." *Child's Nervous System* 27(1), 127-135.

Dincer, A., Yener, U., Özek, M. M. 2011). "Hydrocephalus in patients with neurofibromatosis type 1: MR imaging findings and the outcome of endoscopic third ventriculostomy." *American Journal of Neuroradiology* 32(4), 643-646.

Eguchi, T., Taoka, T., Nikaido, Y., Shiomi, K., Fujimoto, T., Otsuka, H., Takeuchi, H. 1996. "Cine-magnetic resonance imaging evaluation of communication between middle cranial fossa arachnoid cysts and cisterns." *Neurologia medico-chirurgica* 36(6), 353-357.

El Damaty, A., Marx, S., Cohrs, G., Vollmer, M., Eltanahy, A., El Refaee, E., Synowitz, M. 2020. "ETV in infancy and childhood below 2 years of age for treatment of hydrocephalus." *Child's Nervous System* 1-7.

El Gammal, T., Brooks, B. S. 1994. "MR cisternography: initial experience in 41 cases." *American journal of neuroradiology* 15(9), 1647-1656.

Griffiths, P. D., Batty, R., Reeves, M. J., Connolly, D. J. 2009. "Imaging the corpus callosum, septum pellucidum and fornix in children: normal anatomy and variations of normality." *Neuroradiology* 51(5), 337-345.

Hingwala, D., Chatterjee, S., Chandrasekharan Kesavadas, B. T., Kapilamoorthy, T. R. 2011. "Applications of 3D CISS sequence for problem solving in neuroimaging. ." *The Indian journal of radiology & imaging* 21(2), 90.

JPIII, M., Wald, L., Brookeman, J. 2001. "T 2-weighted 3D spin-echo train imaging of the brain at 3 Tesla: reduced power deposition using low flip-angle refocusing RF pulses." *In Proceedings of the 9th annual meeting of ISMRM.* Glasgow, Scotland . 438.

Kim, S. K., Wang, K. C., Cho, B. K. 2000. " Surgical outcome of pediatric hydrocephalus treated by endoscopic III ventriculostomy: prognostic factors and interpretation of postoperative neuroimaging." *Child's Nervous System* 16(3), 161-168.

Kombogiorgas, D., Sgouros, S. 2006. "Assessment of the influence of operative factors in the success of endoscopic third ventriculostomy in children." *Child's Nervous System* 22(10), 1256-1262.

Kulkarni, A. V., Drake, J. M., Armstrong, D. C., Dirks, P. B. 2000. "Imaging correlates of successful endoscopic third ventriculostomy." *Journal of neurosurgery* 92(6), 915-919.

Little, J. R., Houser, O. W., MacCarty, C. S. 1975. "Clinical manifestations of aqueductal stenosis in adults." *Journal of neurosurgery* 43(5), 546- 552.
Lucic, M. A., Koprivsek, K., Kozic, D., Spero, M., Spirovski, M., Lucic, S. 2014. "Dynamic magnetic resonance imaging of endoscopic third ventriculostomy patency with differently acquired fast imaging with steady-state precession sequences." *Bosnian journal of basic medical sciences* 14(3), 165.
Nowosławska, E., Polis, L., Kaniewska, D., Mikołajczyk, W., Krawczyk, J., Szymański, W., Podciechowska. 2003. "Effectiveness of neuroendoscopic procedures in the treatment of complex compartmentalized hydrocephalus in children." *Child's Nervous System* 19(9), 659-665.
Nowosławska, E., Polis, L., Kaniewska, D., Mikołajczyk, W., Krawczyk, J., Szymański, W., Polis, B. 2006. "Neuroendoscopic techniques in the treatment of arachnoid cysts in children and comparison with other operative methods." *Child's Nervous System* 22(6), 599-604.
Oertel, J. M., Schroeder, H. W., Gaab, M. R. 2009. "Endoscopic stomy of the septum pellucidum: indications, technique, and results." *Neurosurgery* 64(3), 482-493.
Osborn, A. G., & Preece, M. T. 2006. "Intracranial cysts: radiologic-pathologic correlation and imaging approach." *Radiology* 239(3), 650-664.
Rakic, P., Yakovlev, P. I. 1968. "Development of the corpus callosum and cavum septi in man." *Journal of Comparative Neurology* 132(1), 45-72.
Rodriguez, J. F., Sosa, F. P., Bustamante, J. L., Lambre, J. P. 2014. *Surgical Treatment Options in Arachnoid Cysts in Children.*
Roth, J., Olasunkanmi, A., Rubinson, K., Wisoff, J. H. 2010. "Septal vein symmetry: implications for endoscopic septum pellucidotomy ." *Operative Neurosurgery* 67(suppl_2), ons395-ons401.
Sarwar, M. 1989. "The septum pellucidum: normal and abnormal." *American Journal of Neuroradiology* 10(5), 989-1005.

Schroeder, H. W., Gaab, M. R. 1999. "Endoscopic aqueductoplasty: technique and results." *Neurosurgery* 45(3), 508-518.

Schroeder, H. W., Oertel, J., & Gaab, M. R. 2004. "Endoscopic aqueductoplasty in the treatment of aqueductal stenosis." *Child's Nervous System* 20(11-12), 821-827.

Schwartz, T. H., Yoon, S. S., Cutruzzola, F. W., Goodman, R. R. 1996. "Third ventriculostomy: post-operative ventricular size and outcome." *min-Minimally Invasive Neurosurgery* 39(04), 122-129.

Tali, E. T., Ercan, N., Kaymaz, M., Pasaoglu, A., Jinkins, J. R. 2004. "Intrathecal gadolinium (gadopentetate dimeglumine enhanced MR cisternography used to determine potential communication between the cerebrospinal fluid pathways and intracranial arachnoid cysts." *Neuroradiology* 46(9), 744-754.

Tubbs, R. S., Oakes, P., Maran, I. S., Salib, C., Loukas, M. 2014. "The foramen of Monro: a review of its anatomy, history, pathology, and surgery." *Child's nervous system* 30(10), 1645-1649.

Udayakumaran, S., Joseph, T. 2019. "Can we predict early endoscopic third ventriculostomy failure? The role of ultra-early postoperative magnetic resonance imaging in predicting early endoscopic third ventriculostomy failure." *World neurosurgery* X, 2, 100013.

Vinas, F. C., Castillo, C., Diaz, F. G. 1998. "Microanatomical considerations for the fenestration of the septum pellucidum." *min-Minimally Invasive Neurosurgery* 41(01), 20-26.

Wang, X., Chen, J. X., You, C., Jiang, S. 2012. "CT cisternography in intracranial symptomatic arachnoid cysts: classification and treatment." *Journal of the neurological sciences* 318(1-2), 125-130.

Yang, D., Korogi, Y., Ushio, Y., Takahashi, M. 2000. "Increased conspicuity of intraventricular lesions revealed by three-dimensional constructive interference in steady state sequences." *American journal of neuroradiology* 21(6), 1070-1072.

Yildiz, H., Erdogan, C., Yalcin, R., Yazici, Z., Hakyemez, B., Parlak, M., Tuncel, E. 2005. "Evaluation of communication between intracranial arachnoid cysts and cisterns with phase-contrast cine MR imaging." *American journal of neuroradiology* 26(1), 145-151.

Chapter 4

ENDOSCOPIC ENDONASAL APPROACH FOR SKULL BASE PATHOLOGIES IN CHILDREN

*Gokmen Kahilogullari**, *MD, PhD*
Ankara University, Department of Neurosurgery, Ankara, Turkey

ABSTRACT

Endoscopic endonasal approach (EEA) has become one of the popular approaches for skull base pathologies (SBP) in children despite the challenges posed by the small size of the developing skull and the narrow endonasal corridors. This review evaluates the efficacy of EEA in the pediatric age group in view of its advantages and disadvantages. Despite the anatomy-related difficulties, the outcomes of EEA are superior owing to its high rate of success and low rate of complications, and the fact that the functional and anatomical integrities of the developing skull and nose of children can be preserved through this approach. EEA is thus an effective and safe approach for treating SBP in children.

---

* Corresponding Author's E-mail: gokmenkahil@hotmail.com.

INTRODUCTION

Skull base pathologies (SBP) vary during the childhood period. Skull base tumors (SBT) are very rarely observed during the childhood and, when present, they are generally benign [9, 25]. Despite being benign and rare, SBT can grow and lead to addition functional loss related to growth, which may prove fatal. Although several operative approaches have been conventionally used for SBP, the endoscopic endonasal approach (EEA) gained popularity in the 2000s not only for adults but also for children [10]. Researches related to the limitations of EEA and to comprehend the red lines for EEA in children are presently the focus of research fields [1, 15, 29, 54].

EEA appears to be a minimally invasive technique owing to its wide visual superiority. This technique continues to develop in the armamentarium of neurosurgeons and otolayrngologists in their efforts to access the ventral skull base as a team [52]. However, considering the minor entrance area in the midline of cranial base lesion in children, it is only possible to reach the lesion from the crista galli to the foramen magnum [25]. Several of the SBP occurring in children can be operated via the EEA. Despite the relative rarity of sellar and anterior skull base lesions in children, EEA remains one of the good options for surgery. SBP can be congenital, tumoral, infectious, traumatic or/and, vascular. The main SBP in children operated with EEA are angiofibromas, craniopharyngiomas, and pituitary tumors. However, some of the other relative pathologies include rhinorrhea (traumatic or spontaneous), meningoencephalocele, Rathke's cleft cyst, chordoma/chordosarcoma, condition related to odontoid pathologies-basilar invagination, gliomas-pilocytic astrocytoma, fibrous dysplasia, hamartoma, neurocytoma, hypophysitis, histiocytosis, abscesses, capillary hemangioma, hemangiopericytoma, dermoid/epidermoid tumors, germinoma, esthesioneuroblastoma, optic nerve decompression, primitive neuroectodermal tumors, and malignancies [5, 9, 11, 16, 19, 20, 23-25, 27, 28, 31, 33, 34, 43, 44-50, 51, 53, 55]. This operative technique is applicable for patients of ages 1 month to 18 years [5, 21, 24, 25, 27, 29, 31, 35, 39].

Anatomical Considerations: Advantages, Disadvantages, and Limitations

The main disadvantages of EEA in children are their small nostrils, narrow corridors, and un-pneumatized sphenoid sinus [24, 30]. Unfavorable anatomical structures in addition to sphenoid pneumatization, the pirifom aperture, and the intercarotid distances are some of the areas that pose potential limitation [52]. Tatreau et al. examined the maxillofacial scans of patients and described that the piriform aperture width was significantly greater in adult patients than in those of age <7 years. In addition, the authors detected that three-fourths of the planum and sellar face and half of the sellar floor were pneumatized in patients aged 6-7 years, and no superior clival pneumatization was evident until the age of 12 years. In their results, clival intercarotid distances did not vary among the different age groups. In fact, they found that the piriforme aperture was possibly a limit only in patients aged <2 years, that sphenoid pneumatization to the planum and sella start at the age of 3 years and complete by the age of 10 years, and that the clival intercarotid distances did not change significantly and were not prohibitively narrow in any of the age groups. Incompletely pneumatized sphenoid sinus required drilling of the bone to access the sellar region, which involved potentially increasing surgery time and theoretically increasing risk of complications [4, 25, 30]. Another limitation for children with EEA is the risk of neurovascular injury, including that to the internal carotid artery, optic nerves or chiasm, or other cranial nerves, which is believed to be largely in part due to the anatomically immature skull base in this age [39, 44, 52]. Kuan et al. stated that there was no significant association between sphenoid pneumatization pattern and the extent of resection, postoperative cerebrospinal fluid (CSF) leak, intraoperative estimated blood loss, total operative time, and the length of stay [30]. In addition, after adjusting for the factors of age, sex, preoperative cranial nerve involvement, and cavernous sinus invasion in their multivariate analyses, they found no significant association among the sphenoid pneumatization pattern and the extent of resection and postoperative CSF leak. No carotid artery or optic nerve injuries as well as no unanticipated intraoperative CSF leaks were encountered in any of the patients in their case series. They defended that sphenoid pneumatization pattern does not appear to affect the outcomes of the EEA in children as well as even in the youngest patients and that the lack of sphenoid pneumatization does not impede the ability to attain gross total resection or increase the perioperative or postoperative complications. With the knowledge of age-related anatomical considerations, some authors emphasized that, in relation to sphenoid pneumatization (developed between the age of 3-10 years), the piriform aperture was significantly smaller in children aged ≤6 years, while the anatomical limit for patients was at age ≤2 years [4, 30, 52]; some studies stated that EEA can be evaluated for younger patients [21, 29, 39]. Kobets et al. described that, with the advancements in the technology of navigation systems, such as thin endoscope equipment, that has lifted the anatomical constraints for infants and young children, EEA seems like a suitable technique with appropriate surgical outcomes [29].

On the other hand, in comparison with the other approaches to skull base, EEA offers some advantages. For instance, Massimi et al. conducted a comparative study between EEA and sublabial microscopic approach in children [38] and found that the rates of admission to the intensive care unit (ICU) were 35% and 100%, the preoperative blood transfusion rates were 23% and 71%, and the postoperative hospital stay durations were 4 days and 5.7 days, respectively. They accordingly added that pain perception was significantly and relatively lower in the EEA group. Therefore, the authors concluded that EEA can improve the quality of the postoperative course in children irrespective of the type of lesions treated and the surgical complications in comparison to the microscopic sublabial approach. Rigante et al. also compared EEA with the conventional microscopic approach in children with the sellar/parasellar region [45]. Based on their results, they assert that the minimal invasiveness makes EEA ideal for the treatment of pediatric lesion of this region, where it is essential to preserve the integrity of the hypothalamic-pituitary axis as well as that of the naso-facial structures in order to assure the correct growth of the child. The transcranial approach is another type of classical surgical approach to the anterior skull base. However, EEA does not require skin incision, external craniotomy, or brain retraction; these advantages are believed to result in significantly fewer complications, faster patient recovery, minimal postoperative discomfort, and reduced overall expense incurred for the treatment [24, 52].

Another debatable issue about EEA is the impact of this technique on the facial and nasal growth zone. Although, theoretically, iatrogenic damage to the nasal growth zones during the childhood period results in mid-facial deformity in the adolescence, although only limited studies have been conducted on the effect of EEA on mid-facial growth with long follow-ups [7, 42]. Parasher et al. compared the craniopharnygioma cases in children operated via the EEA and transcranial approach. They observed that, after 3 years of the surgeries, there were no differences in all cephalometric measurements of mid-facial growth on the follow-up between the two approaches [42]. Chen et al. compared between the 2 groups (n = 44) of children who underwent EEA surgery forvarious pathologies, before the age of 7 years prior to the cranial suture fusion and after the age of 7 years. They found that, although their cohort of patients with skull base lesions demonstrated some abnormal measurements in the maxillary-mandibular relationship before surgeries, their postoperative cephalometric values fell within the normal range at an older age; therefore, there appears to be no evidence of the impact of EEA on craniofacial development within the studied growth period.

Banu et al. described the impact of skull base development on the endoscopic endonasal corridor [3]. They found that skull base development is a slow, gradual, age-dependent, and sex-independent process that can significantly alter the endonasal endoscopic corridors. Thus, preoperative magnetic resonance imaging (MRI) measurements of the skull base are a useful adjunct in selecting the appropriate corridor. The authors also emphasized that the working angles and limits during the dissection or reparative surgery should be measured. Yousseff et al. predicted the limits of the EEA in children and explained the importance of cranial tomography, especially that tailored for craniovertebral junction (CVJ) pathologies [54].

Surgical Preparations and Techniques

In our practice, all children with skull pathologies underwent surgery via the EEA by a panel of neurosurgeons and otolaryngologists who are also members of the endoscopic skull base team. The main advantage of assigning the EAA surgery to this select surgical team was to enable operating the patients with "four hands," "four eyes," and "two minds." In such a situation, it seems that doubling of the philosophy and experience will create a synergy for optimized performance. All patients were assessed at the pediatrics department with their pediatric anaesthiology, pediatric endocrinology, and pediatric oncology teams for patient eligibility for survey and hormonal medications during the preoperative period. If required, postoperative care was provided in the pediatric neurosurgical ICU, and the patients were assessed in the pediatrics department. During the preoperative period, all children underwent MRI and computerized tomography (CT). The tumor size, access rites, bony defects, sinuses, neuromuscular structures, and normal anatomical landmarks with their variations were evaluated by the multidisciplinary surgical team before the surgeries. Mostly, the neuronavigation system was employed to identify the anatomical and pathological structures during the surgery (Figure 1A, 1B, 1C). For navigation, a 1-mm thick sample was subjected to CT and MRI and merged for the system before the surgery [24]. Invasive and eroding skull base lesions can significantly delay the growth of bony structures and affect the relevant measurements; therefore, MRI measurements, rather than age, should ideally guide the preoperative planning scheme [3].

Presently, neurophysiological monitoring is commonly used as an important and useful equipment for these cases [14, 24]. Visual-evoked potentials can be applied in children whose pathology is correlated to the optic nerves and tracts [24] (Figure 1A). Elangovan et al. evaluated the value of intraoperative neurophysiology monitoring (IONM) by electromyography (EMG), brainstem auditory-evoked potentials, and somatosensory-evoked potentials to predict and/or prevent the postoperative neurological deficits for children who underwent EEA for

SBT [14]. They found that IONM can be applied effectively and reliably for these patients and that EMG monitoring is specific for detecting cranial nerve deficits. Accordingly, these tools can serve as effective guide for dissection in these procedures. The authors also added that triggered EMG can be elicited intraoperatively to monitor the integrity of the cranial nerves during and after tumor resection. They believed that, considering the anatomical complexity of EEA in children and the unique challenges encountered therein, multimodal IONM can be a valuable adjunct for these procedures.

The surgical equipment used in these procedures included an 18-cm-long rigid endoscope (diameters: 2.7 mm and 4 mm) with 0-degree optics and a multiangle 4-mm endoscope (Endocameleon Storz, Tuttlingen, Germany) using the 4-hand technique with bilateral nostrils (Figure 1A, 2). Not only the endoscopic equipment systems but also the microneurosurgical instrumentarium, endonasal drill, and the Doppler Systems are kept ready in the operating room. The transnasal transsphenoidal approach is the most common and useful route to reach the sphenoid sinus and anterior fossa. With regards to the surgical stage, the primary surgeon is exchanged with each otolaryngologist and neurosurgeon according to the primary dissection areas below and above the dura mater. In other words, commonly the first half of the surgery is conducted by otolaryngologisy as a primary surgeon with the assistance of neurosurgeon, while the second half witnesses exchange between the surgeons [24]. After the initial exposure to the transnasal corridor, the EEA has 4 corridors for adults or children, as per Kassam et al. [25], which included the transcribriform, transtubercular/transplanum, transpolar, and transclival corridors located along the rostrocaudal axis. The transcribriform approach extends the previous exposure rostrally to the level of the crista galli. If required, this approach may be combined with the Draf III procedure (frontal sinusotomy) to reach the back wall of the frontal sinus. As an advantage of this approach, the anterior and posterior ethmoidal arteries can be identified and, if necessary, coagulated at the beginning of the tumor and removed for tumor revascularization. The removal of the crista galli and cribriform plate provides a large space for better surgical condition in the anterior frontal fossa from the frontal sinus to the planum sfenoidale and in the lateral line to the lamina papyracea. This approach may be useful for the pathologies of anterior skull base, such as traumatic CSF leakage and fibro-osseous tumor esthesioneuroblastoma, in children. The transtubercular/transplanum approach allows reaching to the supresellar area without violating the sella. This approach is especially useful in cases where the sella is not expanded from its normal size. However, the transtubercular/transplanum approach can combined with the transsellar exposure when required. One of the advantages of this approach is that the olfactory structures can be protected, because the intervention does not extend rostrally to the posterior ethmoidal arteries. This approach may be useful in SBP of this region and suprasellar pathologies such as suprasellar craniopharyngiomas, giant pituitary adenoma, traumatic CSF leakage, meningocele, and fibro-osseous tumor in children. The transsellar approach is the most commonly applied approach with EEA in children, considering the high rates of pathologies in this area. In this approach, the planum tuberculum and bilaterally lamina papyraccea are exposed and the floor of the sphenoid sinus is drilled back to the clivus. This approach may be useful for the sellar/parasellar pathologies such as craniopharyngioma, pituitary adenoma, and Rathke's cleft cyst (RCC) in children. The transclivus approach is rarely applied with the EEA for children. The clivus extends from the dorsum sella to the foramen magnum. This approach may be useful to treat clival pathologies such as traumatic cordoma/ chordosarcoma, fibro-osseous tumor, and odontoidectomy in children [4, 25, 49].

For older children, after the placement of adrenalin-impregnated cottonoids for controlling mucosal bleeding and widening the operative corridor, the middle turbinate was lateralized, the posterior septum was removed, the sphenoid ostiums were bilaterally enlarged, and the sphenoid sinuses were exposed after the removal of the rostrum of the nasal septum, which allowed the application of "two nostrils four hands technique." After operative visualization of the bony landmarks that guide and orient surgeons to the midline and pathology, the seller floor was removed, and the dura was exposed and opened. Following the microsurgical principles, tumor debunking and cytoreduction were performed, and the dissection plane between the tumor and normal vital structures was visualized and controlled, after which the tumor was sharply dissected from the surrounding tissues based on its adhesiveness and stiffness [41].

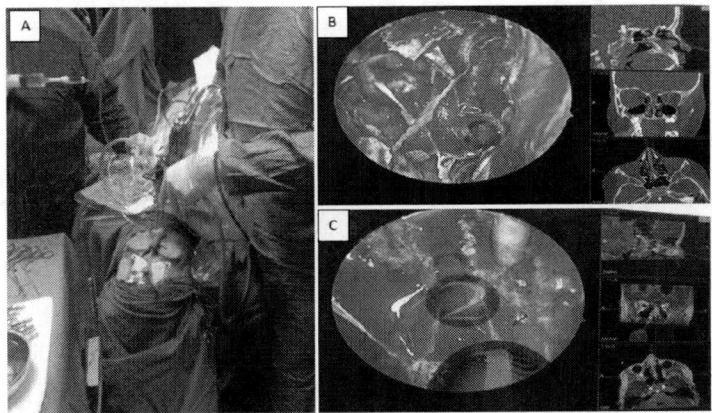

Figure 1. Neuronavigation and visual evoked potential noromonitarization system in a patient operated via EEA (A), neuronavigation system with CT (B) and MRI (C) confirmations.

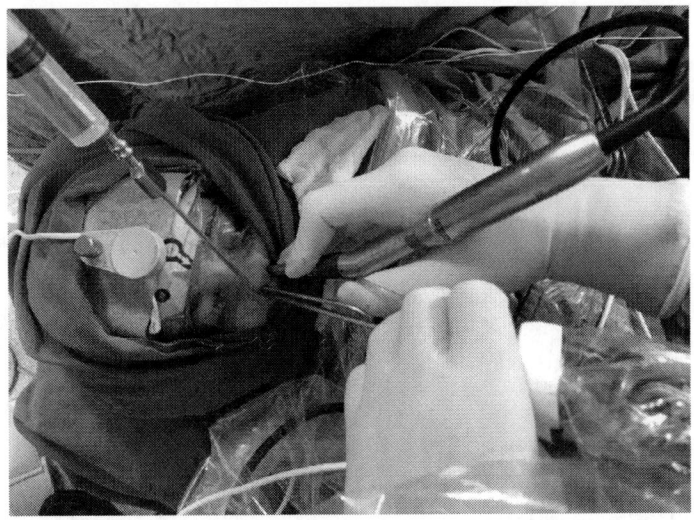

Figure 2. Endoscopic surgical tools operated via EEA in a child.

Owing to the anatomical specifications presented in younger children and infants, such as small nostrils and unpneumatizated sphenoid sinuses, appropriate instrumentation and techniques along with enhanced technical knowledge is utilized. Tools that are smaller in size and appropriate for atraumatic techniques were used to combat the issue of the small nostrils. Bone drilling was next performed for resculpturing and creating artificial sphenoid sinuses in the unpneumatizated samples and for the surgical procedure. For patients who were operated for rhinorrhea and/or meningocele/meningoencephalocele diagnosed on a comprehensive algorithm, a preoperative intrathecal sodium fluorescein injection was administered from the lumbar site to enable intraoperative CSF tracking on the night before the surgery [24].

Commonly, the patients were admitted to the ICU on the first day of surgery; however, in cases of cranial complications such as hemorrhage, serious electrolyte imbalance, long surgery times, and long-duration anesthesia, this time can be longer. The mean hospital stay of the patients operated by the EEA was 4.4 days [24].

Pathologies

Some of the common and rare SBP operated with the EEA are presented below. Considering the debate of angiofibromas that it is SBP or nasopharyngeal pathologies, angiofibromas were not included in this section.

Craniopharyngioma

Craniopharygiomas are well-known benign, often calcified and/or cystic and occasionally behaviorally aggressive tumors, and EEA is one of most useful approach for craniopharygiomas during the childhood period [2, 24, 41, 43]. Over one-third of craniopharygiomas are detected in the pediatric population, and they account for 10% of all pediatric intracranial tumors [43]. The patient may present with increased intracranial pressure signs, hydrocephalus, and visual problems related to the mass effect on chiasma opticum and hypothalamic-pituitary dysfunctions. Of the numerous surgical approaches known, the EEA has gained much popularity in the recent years [41]. In most of the series, craniopharyngiomas were reported as the most common pathology among children operated by the EEA [9, 11, 16, 24, 28]. Whether gross total resection or subtotal resection with adjuvant radiotherapy is better for craniopharyniomas remains controversial [43]. Although, these are debatable issues, total resection is considered to be safer with little complication risk and is usually the target of surgical intervention. In the past 2 decades, as for all the other sellar lesions, EEA is increasingly being preferred as the surgical approach for craniopharyngioma in children [2, 24, 43]. In our past study, we compared the EEA and open microscopic transcranial approaches for patients of all ages with craniopharyngioma and suggested the EEA as the first-line of surgical treatment modality in patients with a preliminary diagnosis of craniopharyngioma in terms of low complication risk, minimal invasiveness, and better outcome scores [41]. We thus suggested that open microscopic transcranial procedures may be combined with the EEA in a single session for challenging cases. Chivucula et al. reported that the total resection rate for craniopharyngioma 18-76% as per the literature and that its success rate depends on the tumor size and approach [9]. In their case series of 16 pediatric craniopharyngiomas cases of the EEA, Patel et al. noted a gross total resection rate of 93.8%, and majority of the patients (66.7%) presenting the symptoms were resolved in the early postoperative period [43]. However, new incidences of panhypopituitarism have been reported in 63.6% and that of diabetes insipid in 46.7% of the patients. The major complication rate was 12.5%, and the CSF leak rate was 18.8% in this case series. The authors reported that 1 patient died from intraventricular hemorrhage (6.3%) and the disease recurred in another 1 patient (6.3%). Based on their experience, the authors concluded that, although EEA is an extremely effective approach for craniopharyngioma in the childhood period with a high rate of total resection and a low rate of disease recurrence, where hypothalamic-pituitary disfunction and CSF leak continue to remain significant postoperative morbidities (Figure 3).

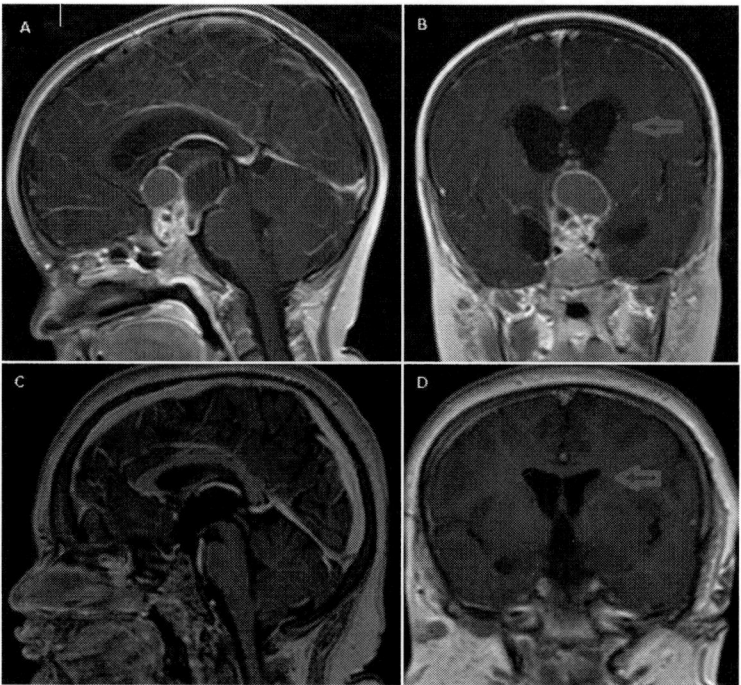

Figure 3. A 7-year-old boy with craniopharyngioma operated via the EAA. Preoperative coronal (A) and sagittal (B) and postoperative fifth years coronal (C) and sagittal (D) MRI sections. Total resection achieved. Lateral ventricul dilatation has improved by the years due to operation (red arrows, B and D).

Pituitary Adenoma

Pediatric pituitary adenomas are rare lesions, and their incidence in the childhood brain tumors is reportedly 1-10% [32]. Despite the rarity of pituitary adenomas, alterations in the hormone functions may cause a significant effect on the quality-go-life. It is one of the benign tumor that can be treated via surgical intervention and correction of any related hormone deficiency, if required medically. Despite the practice of the transcranial and/or transsphenoidal approaches, EEA has recently become a preferable approach for the treatment of pituitary adenomas during the childhood [9, 24, 34]. Chivukula et al. described that, overall, the rate of total tumor was 90% in their case series for secretory adenomas, and these rates reportedly ranged 40-80% in the literature [9]. Locatelli et al. conducted a multi-center retrospective study on 27 pediatric patients, which included 12 patients (48.14%) with the Cushing's disease, 5 (18.5%) with growth hormone-secreting adenoma, 5 (18.5%) with prolactinoma, and 4 (14.8%) with non-functional adenoma; of these patients, 81.4% met the remission criteria, but 18.5% did not [34]. The authors thus concluded that despite the practice of EEA or microscopic approach, the transsphenoidal resection in of adenomas remain the mainstay treatment with proven cure in the pediatric ages; moreover, the personal experience of the performing neurosurgeon designates the choice of treatment.

Pituitary adenomas are generally the second-most commonly presenting SBP in the case series of children operated by the EEA [11, 16, 24] (Figure 4).

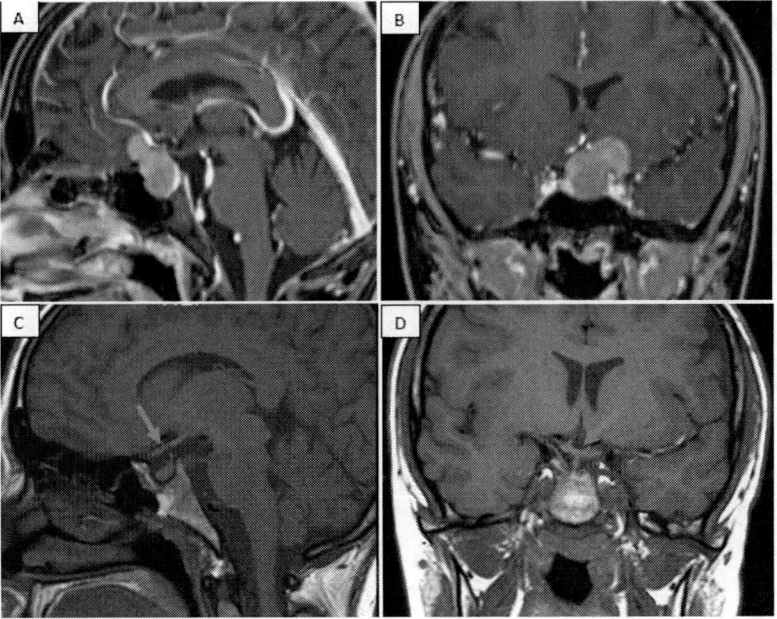

Figure 4. A 9-year-old girl with pituitary adenoma operated via the EAA. Preoperative coronal (A) and sagittal (B) and postoperative coronal (C) and sagittal (D) MRI sections. Total resection achieved. Optic chiasm (blue arrows, C and D) and pituitary gland-stalk (red arrows, C and D) are decompressed after operation.

Ratkhe's Cleft Cyst (RCC)

The RCC are benign lesions derived from the Ratkhe's pouch. They are usually detected in the seller or suprasellar area. Although they have extremely high rates of detection in autopsy, RCC was commonly diagnosed incidentally, and only <10% of the patients presented with any symptoms. These incidences were lower in children than in adults [37, 48]. In the case of symptomatic RCC, primary surgery with the EEA was preferred not only for adults but also for children [37, 49]. Shepard et al. examined 24 pediatric patients with RCC, of whom 7 were operated with the EEA and 17 were managed conservatively [48]. In the operated 7 patients, 3 patients showed the complication of transient Diabetes insipidus (DI) and 1 showed adrenal insufficiency. Only 1 case of recurrence occurred. The authors thus concluded that, like adults, in RCC children may exhibit spontaneous growth and shrinkage. The authors also suggested that, in case of optic nerve compression without visual deterioration and/or when the diagnosis is uncertain, this pathology can be managed conservatively.

Interestingly, in the largest two series of SBP operated with EAA, RCC has been described as the second-most common SBP among children who were operated with the EEA [9, 28].

Chordoma

Chordoma is a low-grade, aggressive tumor that has a high recurrence risk. Generally, this tumor is located midline, especially, in the sacrum and clivus. Surgery is extremely important for treating chordomas, because of the recurrence risk and because the prognosis is related to the surgical success. In addition, EEA is the preferred surgical technique for these cases owing to the high success rate and low complication rate of EEA in comparison to other surgical techniques not only for adults but also for children [17, 56]. Chivucula et al. explained that, the total rate of chordoma occurrence is 4.7-58% in the literature, with the application of diverse approaches across different ages groups [9]. However, in their series for children, the total resection rate was 50% for chordoma cases. The authors stated that, although complete resection remains the surgical target, this target must be tempered by an understanding of the need for other treatment options such as radiotherapy and/or chemotherapy and the overall quality-of-life outcome.

Despite it being rare among the pediatric group, Shenouda et al. reported 29 cases of pediatric chordoma that were operated with the EEA in their meta analyses [47].

Craniovertebral Junction Pathologies (CVJ)

The EEA to the pediatric CVJ is a relatively new technique that provides an alternative to the transoral approach to the anterior pediatric spine and CVJ pathologies [20, 22, 25, 51]. Kassam et al. stated that it is possible to reach EEA below C-2 with the EEA in the sagittal plane, not only in adults but also in children [25]. Access to the CVJ can be extremely challenging owing to the complex anatomy of this region, and the conventional transoral approach is widely recognized as the standard procedure, despite its limitations and drawbacks [51]. These limitations can be predicted on the basis of radiological and anatomical measurements and the knowledge about the pediatric population [54]. Youssef et al. explained that the caudal limit of the EEA extends to as far as the middle-third of the odontoid process in children, as predicted by the nasoaxial line, and they found that the length of the plate was a significant predictor of the working distance to C-2. They accordingly concluded that the preoperative utilization of the nasoaxial line may help plan EEA to the CVJ in children. Although, presently EEA has become more popular, only a few cases have been reported that too with a small number of patients in the literature [20, 51]. The indications for EEA in CVJ pathologies occurred with Chiari malformation, basilar invagination, spinal cord compression in CVJ, and retroflexed odontoid process [20, 22, 51]. After EEA decompression of CVJ, subsequent posterior decompression and fusion may be required [20, 22, 25, 51]. Despite its known effectiveness, EEA in children with CVJ pathologies may be associated with some issues. For instance, Tan et al. noted that 1 of 3 cases in their series required long-term tracheostomy care although all patients were allowed oral intake within a week and discharged in good condition [47]. In our previous case report with the

EEA approach for CVJ pathologies in children, we recorded a pneumocephalus complication after EEA odontoidectomy in a patient who fully recovered a week after the second EEA reconstruction surgery [20]. It seems that the EEA to the CVJ provides a potentially safer alternative in the pediatric population, warranting future studies with large series size to analyze the validity of this novel technique [51].

Meningoencephalocele/Cephalocele

Meningoencephalocele/cephalocele (M/C) in relation to the skull base is rare and majority of them are congenital lesions manifesting as nasal masses requiring surgical intervention in children. M/C could be congenital or developed due to trauma. EEA is a preferable approach for these patients and applicable for children all of all ages from newborns to adolescents [5, 8, 24, 26, 38]. These pathologies are deemed to be meningoencephalocele when the sac contains no neural elements and as encephalocele when the sac contains it. Pediatric M/C has been conventionally addressed with the transcranial approaches owing to its high complication rate resulting from brain retractions, high hemorrhage volumes, and potentially epilepsy situation. Although some authors maintain that M/C can never be managed by a transnasal approaches alone, several recent studies have described the superiority of EEA in these pathologies [8, 11, 26]. The repair of M/C by the EEA reconstruction technique has become more effective and present with lower rhinorrhea risks [5, 24, 36]. These reconstruction techniques, such as nasoseptal flap (NF), can be used even in very young children with M/C, as also reported earlier [5]. In relation to past studies and surgical outcomes, this opinion is justifiable that the EEA is a preferred surgical approach for M/C during the childhood period in comparison with the conventional surgeries owing to its minimally invasive concept, cosmesis, efficiency, shorter hospital stay, safer procedure, and affordability of the treatment.

Reconstruction-Nasoseptal Flap (NF)

Reconstruction and repairing are extremely important parts of EEA for patients of all ages, because of its most-criticized limitation of the potential rhinorrhea risk. EEA is preferable over open surgery because it requires no external incision or craniotomy, and it is associated with lower rates of neurological complications and lower costs of the procedure in comparison to those of the transcranial surgery. However, on the other hand, an extremely important and common complication is of rhinorrhea that occurs in 3.5-23% of all affected children operated with EEA [40]. EEA is being increasingly used for the reconstruction and repairing of SBP [5, 6, 12, 13, 18, 32, 36, 39, 40, 46]. With the common usage of vascularized-pedicled NF (Hadad Flap) for the required cases in EEA, the rhinorrhea rates decreased significantly in adults and children with SBP [5, 6, 13, 24, 25, 46]. With the multilayer reconstruction technique and with the use of vascularized NF, rate of rhinorrhea occurrence can be reduced to as low as 5% [6, 24, 25]. Ben-Ari et al. described that the use of NF is both an effective and a safe technique for the reconstruction of skull base defects and pathologies in children owing its high success and low complication rate. The authors also added that there was no apparent negative influence on the cranifacial growth in their series through this approach [6]. Shah et al. stated that NF may not be a viable option for EEA reconstruction in children aged <10 years, with reliable option in patients aged >14 years; moreover, patients aged 10-13 years require careful consideration of facial analysis and preoperative radio anatomic evaluation on an individual basis [46]. Conversely, some authors defend that the use of NF is not related to the age of the patient directly and can hence be used effectively for children of all ages (even infants) [5, 12, 13, 18, 36, 39]. In our previous case series, we reported that 50% of the 54 patients showed intraoperative CSF leakage; however, only 1 patient had rhinorrhea after the postoperative period, who underwent the repair process during the second surgery [24]. In this series, NF was used in 26 patients who required multilayer reconstruction techniques with no lumbar drainage. Interestingly, for the very young cases, Nation et al. described that, even in 50% of the patients with CSF leaks during the intraoperative period, zero patients experienced postoperative CSF leak by the reconstruction techniques [39]. The EEA skull base reconstruction techniques, in addition to the use of vascularized flaps for dural and bone defects, nonvascularized flaps for dural and bone defects, and for complex defects free-tissue transfer techniques can be used [13]. Di Rocco et al. suggested that even when compared with the external subfrontal approach, the EEA seems to be a less risky; in extremely large defects or when the defects extend too far anteriorly or laterally, a combined EEA and subfrontal approach may be better [12]. Ma et al. emphasized the importance of preoperative imaging by CT and MRI for the detection of the defect site and for selecting the appropriate operative approach and the appropriate reconstructive graft material along with skilled surgeon/s and the surgical team with experience in EEA [36]. The endoscopic endonazal approach for treating skull base defects and/or for SBP is it's a commonly used technique owing to its minimally invasive nature, efficiency, safety with low complications, and a high success rates in children (Figure 5).

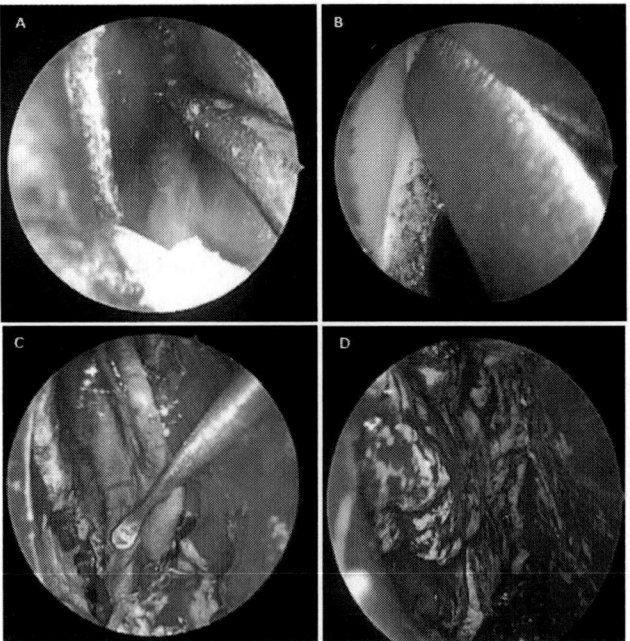

Figure 5. The preparation and using of nasoseptal flap in a child operated via EEA; the bordering the line of flap with unipolar cautery (A), the dissection of flap from the cartilage tissue (B), after dissection ready-to-use pedunculed and vascularized flap (C), completely covering the constructed area with nasoseptal flap (D).

Miscellaneous

There are some rare SBP that are operated via the EEA and presented in series and/or published as case reports, which include fibro-osseus tumors, chordoma/chordosarcoma, germinoma, hypothalamic/optic gliomas, pilocytic astrositomas, schwannoma, esthesioneuroblastoma, dermoid/epidermoid tumors, pontin cavernoma, capillary hemangioma, clival arteriovenous malformation (AVM), hemangioperistoma, neurocytoma, hypophysitis, langerhans histiocytosis, hamartomas, rhabdoid tumor/teratoma, meningiomas, inverted papilloma, lymphoma, cholesterol granuloma, ependymoma, osteoma, leiomyoma, abscesses, optic nerve decompressions, and malign/metastatic tumors [9, 11, 16, 19, 23-25, 27, 47, 50, 53] (Figure 6-9).

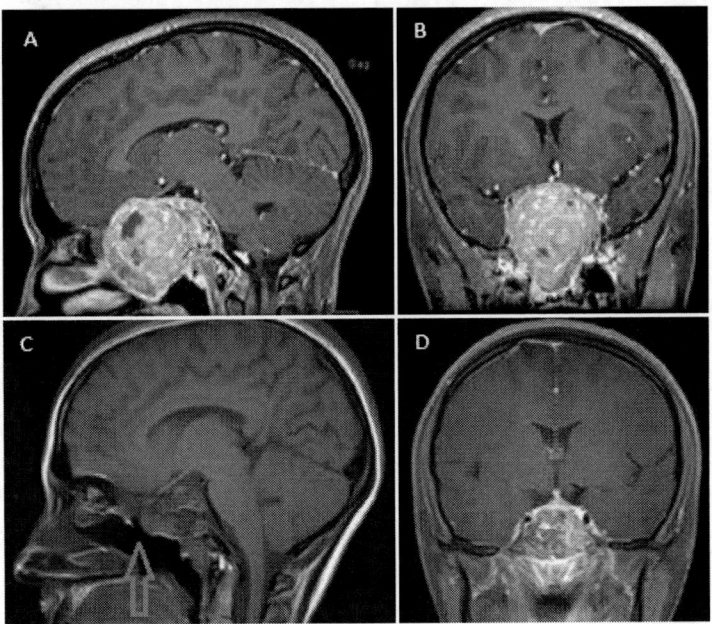

Figure 6. A 14-year-old girl with giant cell bone tumor operated via the EEA. Preoperative coronal (A) and sagittal (B) and postoperative coronal (C) and sagittal (D) MRI sections. Total resection achieved. It appears that the previously closed airline has been completely opened (blue arrow, C).

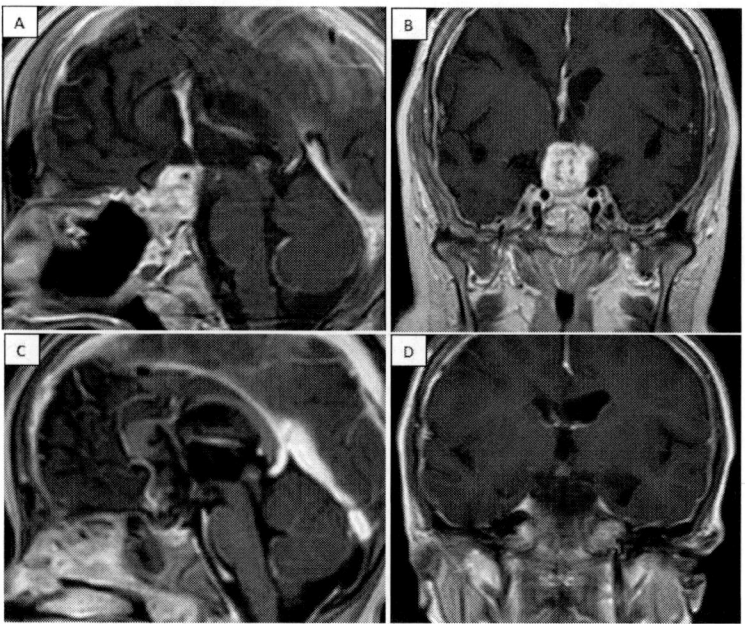

Figure 7. A 12-year old girl with pilocytic astrositoma operated via the EEA. Preoperative coronal (A) and sagittal (B) and postoperative coronal (C) and sagittal (D) MRI sections. Total resection achieved.

Benign fibro-osseous tumors can be located in the skull base in children and can be related to the surrounding anatomical structures such as the nasal cavity, paranasal sinuses, nasal cavity, and orbit. The surgical removal and pathological diagnosis are extremely important and required for these tumors. Stapleton et al. presented a case series of 14 children operated with the EEA from Pittsburgh [50]. They recorded that of all the patients, 6 had juvenile ossifying fibroma, 5 had benign fibro-osseous lesion, 2 had osteoma, and 1 had fibrous dysplasia. Overall, 10 patients achieved gross total resection in this series, and there were no cases of postoperative CSF leaks or any other major complications. The authors describe that EEA is a safe and effective treatment for benign fibro-osseous tumors of the skull base in children (Figure 6).

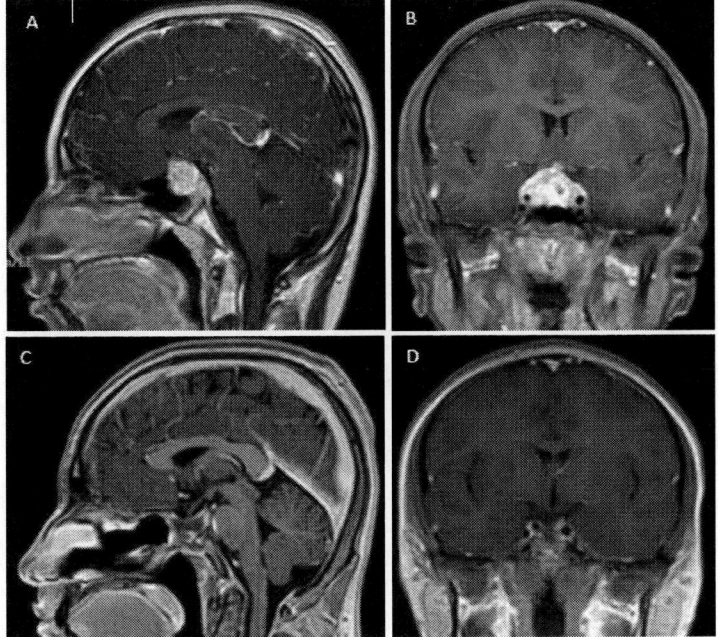

Figure 8. A 13-year old boy with poorly differentiated malignant epithelial tumor operated via the EEA. Preoperative coronal (A) and sagittal (B) and postoperative fourth years coronal (C) and sagittal (D) MRI sections. No residual tumor left after additional chemotherapy and radiotherapy.

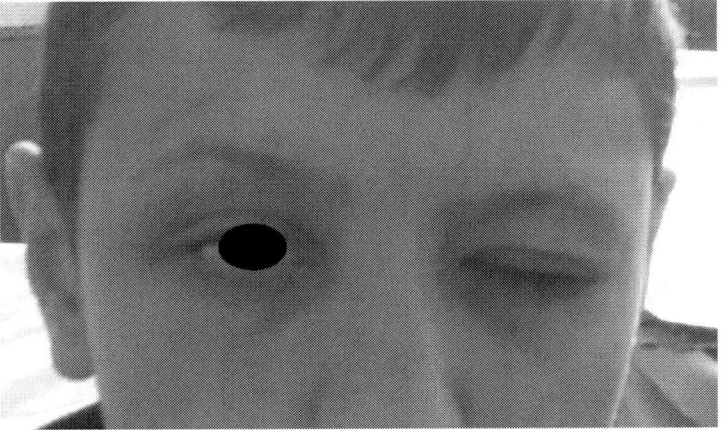

Figure 9. Left-sided total ophtalmoplegia due to cavernous sinus invasion in the child in Figure 8.

Dermoid cysts/tumors are true ectodermal inclusion cyst accounting for approximately 0.3% of all intracranial tumors. Generally, they arise in the midline and are congenital, benign lesions. Sellar dermoid tumors are extremely rare and reported only in 17 cases, which included 4 children; we had previously reported these cases in a review of the literature [23]. The EEA may be considered as the first choice in eligible patients for the skull base and the sellar/parasellar lesions, including in pediatric cases. Another extremely rare pathology of the skull base in children is embryonal tumors. Sellar and skull base embryonal tumors are exceedingly rare, with only 13 cases reported so far and only 3 pediatric cases, which we had previously presented as a review of the literature with a unique pediatric case operated via the EEA [53]. Notably, these very rare tumors are diagnosed by biopsy and histology and can be treated by adjuvant radio/chemotherapy, making the EEA appropriate in such pediatric cases.

Optic nerve fenestration via the EEA is one of the rarely operative approach in children who suffer from idiopathic hypertension (pseudotumor cerebri). In this pathology, intracranial pressure is increased without any evident clinical or radiological findings with the normal CSF constituents. Cases with visual loss problems and the decompression of the optic nerve with the transcranial or transnasal routes require operative approaches. Although this situation is very rarely observed in children, recently, endoscopic optic nerve decompression has become the preferred surgical approaches for this age group. Gupta et al. presented 15 children who were diagnosed with pseudo tumor cerebri and operated with optic nerve decompression via EEA [19]. The authors found that 13 of the 15 patients experienced reversal of vision loss, and only 2 children did not show any improvement because of their optic atrophy history. The authors explained that, in the follow-up period, none of the patients showed any recurrence. As a relatively new surgical option, optic nerve decompression via the EEA is a minimally invasive approach and an effective alternative to prevent vision loss in comparison with other surgical approaches for idiopathic intracranial hypertension in children.

Series/Meta-analysis

Because of the increased popularity and as a preferable approach, EEA for sellar/parasellar regions [33, 55] and SBP in children have been published by several case series [4, 9, 11, 16, 24, 25, 27, 28] in the past decades and also in recent meta-analysis [31, 47].

Zhan et al. presented the retrospective analysis of 11 pediatric patients of age >2 years who underwent EEA for the resection of the sellar region [55]. They described that all patients had pituitary adenoma, 8 patients had macro-adenoma and 3 had microadenomas. The total resection rate was 81.8%, and the subtotal resection rate was 18.2%; no patient showed partial or insufficient resection. All patients achieved visual remission (100%), and 7 of the 8 patients (87.5%) with the hyperhormone levels in preoperative evaluation experienced endocrinological remission in the postoperative period. Three patients, (27.3%) of the patients required hormone replacement in the postoperative period for newly developed hypopituitarism, and and two patients (18.2%) developed temporary diabetes inspidus. One patient incurred postoperative CSF leakage that resolved after lumbar drainage, and there were no cases of meningitis, intracranial hematoma, or death in their series.

Locatelli et al. described 27 children who were operated with the EEA, of which 17 had sellar, 7 suprasellar, and 3 clival pathologies [33]. They stated that all the surgeries were performed by a team of a neurosurgeon and an otolaryngologist. The total resection rate was 81.5%, while the subtotal resection rate was 7.5% and partial removal rate was 11%. Pituitary adenoma was the most common pathology (n = 12 patients), followed by craniopharyngioma (n = 5) and RCC (n = 4). Postoperative CSF leakage occurred in 3 patients; in 2 cases, it occurred after multilayer reconstruction surgery and in 1 patient after transient limber drainage, but the problem was resolved. Preoperative hypopituitarism disappeared or improved in 4 cases and became stable in the remaining 2 patients in their series. The authors stated that no neurological morbidity or mortality was noted after the surgery.

The team of Kassam et al. is the pioneer team in the Pittsburgh Group who published one of the first series on the EEA for SBP in adults as well as in children. In 2007, they published a children series with skull base lesions who were operated fully by the EEA [25]. In their series of 25 children, there were 4 patients with Cushing syndrome, 3 each with juvenile nasal angiofibroma and fibro-osseus lesion, 2 each with prolactinoma, germinoma, and RCC, and 1 patient each with epidermoid tumor, lymphoma, optic nerve glioma, neuroendocrin tumor, chroma, hypertrophic pituitary gland, optic nerve decompression, clival AVM, and CSF leakage. Interestingly, no craniopharyngioma cases were noted in this series, although it is one of most common pathology with a high number of reporting recently. The gross total resection was 80%, and the most-frequently described condition was CSF leakage in 2 patients (8%). No case of meningitis, serious morbidity, or death occurred in their series. Kassam et al. demonstrated the feasibility of performing EEA to access the midline cranial base lesions from the crista galli to the foramen magnum for a wide variety of lesions from AVMs to tumors in this one of the first series from this area. They estimated that the addition of visualization and exposure would provide comparable outcomes by resection to those attained with the transcranial or transracial approaches.

Khalili et al. published 27 cases of children with skull base diseases who were operated via the EEA [27]. In their series, the most common pathology was craniopharyngioma (n = 13), followed by pituitary lesion, chordoma, germinoma, RCC, optic glioma, and encephalocele with 2 cases each and by hamartoma and rhabdoid tumor with 1 case each. Banu et al. presented 33 pediatric patients in their series and reported the most common pathology of craniopharyngioma and angiofibroma with 5 patients each, followed by prolactinoma, pituitary apoplexy, and CSF leakage/meningoencephalocele with 4 patients each [4]. The authors explained that their gross total resection was 75%. In their series, significant improvement was noted in 58.3% of the patients with visual deficits. There was no case of rhinorrhea, albeit there were 5% of infection rate, without death. The authors emphasized the importance of radianatomical skull base measurements for the predicted complications, which they stated to be more important than age. Giovanetti et al. presented 44 pediatric cases with SBP that were operated with the EEA

[16]. In this series, the most commonly pathologies were craniopharyngioma and pituitary adenoma. They noted 3 main postoperative complications, namely, rhinorrhea in 2 patients and cerebral abscess in 1 patient. They also described the importance of the use of vascularized NF for skull base reconstruction, which reduced the rate of postoperative CSF leakage. In a recent study presented by Deopujari et al. on 49 children [11], the most commonly pathology was craniopharyngioma (n = 22) and pituitary adenoma (n = 8). The authors explained that the goal of surgery achieved in 47 out of 49 patients. In 2 patients, transient DI developed, which later resolved. The authors observed CSF leakage during surgery but managed the leak with lumbar drainage. Rhinorrhea occurred in 3 patients. One patient with craniopharyngioma expired due to ventriculitis.

Over the 50 patients there are three series in the literature [9, 24, 28]. In our previously published series, we presented 54 patient who underwent an operation by an endoscopic skull base team comprising of neurosurgeons and an otolaryngologist. Craniopharyngioma (29.6%) was most commonly pathology detected, followed by pituitary adenoma (22.2%) in this series. Cases with angiofibromas were excluded from the series. The gross total resection rate was 76.7%; however, the subtotal resection was achieved in 16.2% and 6.9% patients with the primary goal of being able to conduct biopsy for histopathological examination. Of all, 11 patients showed postoperative transient DI and 2 showed craniopharyngioma with a temporary loss of vision, which completely improved within a week after surgery. Only 1 patient who was operated with basilar invagination developed postoperative rhinorrhea and pneumocephalus, although no CSF leakage was detected during the first surgery and in those who were reconstructed in the second surgery [22, 24]. One patient showed panhypopituitarism related to the surgery. This patient had visual acuity loss before surgery, while 35.1% of all patients showed improvement due to decompression of the optic nerves. This series is a unique study of children of all age groups with respect to their pathologies and the olfaction status in preoperative and postoperative period presented in this series. The olfaction status results revealed 31.4%

rate in a patient with a sleigh loss of olfactory functions after surgery. The loss was scored from 1 to 8 points in all patients, except for one, who recovered completely after 6 months of the surgery. No changes or improvements in the olfactory functions were observed in 68.5% of all patients. Notably, CSF leak was detected in half of the cases; however, only 1 case of rhinorrhea was recorded in the follow-up. Despite the high rate of CSF leak in the perioperative period, the very low rate of rhinorrhea can be explained by the use of pedicled NF and multilayer reconstruction techniques with effectivity during the childhood period. No mortality was occurred during the perioperative period; however, one patient with craniopharyngioma died from hormonal and electrolyte imbalance at the end of the second week of surgery [24].

Kim et al. reported that a huge number of children presenting only with brain tumors were operated via the endoscopic endonasal skull base surgery (28). The most common tumors in them included craniopharyngioma (n = 39), followed by RCC (n = 15), pituitary adenoma (n = 13), germinoma (n = 8), chordoma (n = 3), langerhans cell histiocytosis (n = 2), and others (n = 2). The gross total resection rate was 90.9%. All patients with craniopharyngioma, pituitary adenoma, and chordoma underwent gross total resection even if they were primary or recurrent cases. In this series, the vision improvement was 76.1%, however the endocrinological status improved only in 10 patients. The CSF leakage rate was 2.4% and only observed in 2 patients operated for RCC. Aseptic meningitis or bacterial meningitis was the most common complication (7.3%) in this series, and one case of delayed intraventricular hemorrhage was also reported in a patient operated for craniopharyngioma; despite the emergent craniotomy in this patient, severe sequelae remained in this patient.

The largest series in the literature was published by Chivukula from Pittsburgh with 133 patients, including 112 with SBT and 21 with bony lesions [9]. Moreover, the series included 32 patients with angiofibriomas, 16 with craniopharyngiomas, 12 with RCC, 11 with pituitary adenoma, 10 with chordorma/chondrosarcomas, 9 with dermoid/epidermoid tumors, and 30 with other pathologies. The gross total resection rates for this pathology were 76.2% for angiofibromas, 56.2% for craniopharyngiomas, 72.7% for RCC, 70% for pituitary adenoma, 50% for chordoma/chordosarcoma, 85.7% for dermoid/epidermoid tumors, and 31% for other pathologies. In 15.4% of all patients, recurrence occurred, and the patients underwent re-surgery. Vascularized NF was used in 55 patients, intranasal balloon in 19 patients as a reconstruction technique, autologous fat graft in 14 patients, free mucosal graft in 10 patients, and vascularized pericardial flap in 1 patient. The CSF leakage rate was 10.5%, meningitis accounted for 3.8%, transient DI for 6%, permanent DI for 9%, transient cranial nerve palsies for 3.8%, and permanent cranial nerve palsies for 2.3% as complications.

Some past meta analyses have been published about EEA in children for SBP [31, 47]. For instance, Lee et al. searched the PubMed, Scopus, and Cochrane Library in their meta-analysis and shortlisted 25 articles with 554 patients for the seller and suprasellar lesions [31]. They reviewed only 3 pathologies of this region, which included craniopharyngioma, pituitary adenomas, and RCC. The mean age of the patients was 11.3 years, with male:female ratio of 1.4/1. The most common pathology was the craniopharyngioma (52%), followed by pituitary adenoma (33%) and RCC (13%). The gross total resection was 77.6%, and specific to pathology resection rate was 75.8% for craniopharyngioma, 81.8% for pituitary adenoma, and 69.7% for RCC. The overall CSF leakage was described as 8.6%; however, the pathology specific rates were 10.6% for craniopharyngioma, 6.5% for pituitary adenoma, and 7.2% for RCC. The authors found that postoperative CSF leakages were significantly greater in the younger children than in the older children. The other complications included meningitis (3.4%), obesity/weight gain (3.4%), vascular injury (1.9%), and cranial nerve palsy (1.5%). The baseline diabetes insipidus was observed to be greater in craniopharyngioma (24%) than in pituitary adenoma (1.2%) and RCC (9.3%). The postoperatively new permanent DI occurred in approximately half of the craniopharyngioma cases (51.1%), followed by that in pituitary adenoma cases (4.3%) and in RCC (6.6%). Preoperative hypopituitarism occurred in greater number pituitary adenoma cases (69.1%), and comparatively lower in craniopharyngioma cases (57.1%) and in RCC cases (28.1%). The best improvement was observed in the pituitary adenoma group (83.7%), followed by that in the craniopharyngioma cases (8.3%). New postoperative hypopituitarism cases occurred in 46.6% of all patients, but the highest rate was recorded in craniopharyngioma cases (71.3%) and in pituitary adenoma cases (21.9%) and RCC cases (12.5%). The highest visual deficit rate was noted in patients presenting with craniopharyngioma (57.4%), followed by those presenting with pituitary adenoma (33.8%) and then RCC (31.5%). The best improvement occurred in RCC cases (96.1%), followed by pituitary adenoma cases (79%) and craniopharyngioma cases (75.6%). Permanent visual deficit occurred in 2.6% of all patients, with similar rates in the other 3 pathologies. Shenouda et al. shortlisted 93 studies including 574 patients from the search on the PubMed/MEDLINE, Cochtan Library Embase, and Web of Science database [47]. The average age of the patients was 12.8 years (range: newborn to 18 years) in this meta-analysis, with male patients being distinctly more than female patients (72% versus 27%). The gross total resection rate was 58% and the subtotal resection was 14%, but the unspecified resection rate from the series was 19%. The recurrence rates were 12.5% and the average rate for recurrence was approximately 20 months. Juvenil nasopharyngeal angiofibroma was the most common pathology with 41.6% recurrence rate, followed by craniopharyngioma (15.5%) and pituitary adenoma (9.1%). Chondrosarcomas has been described as the most common malignant pathologies (1.9%), followed by sarcomas (0.7%). Nasopharynx (18.6%) and suprasellar location (14.9%) are the most common locations of all central SBT. The most common sign and symptoms explained were nasal obstruction (16.5%), headache (16%), endocrinopathy (14.3%), and epistaxis (14%). The most common early complications (occurring before 6 weeks of surgery) were CSF leak (17.3%), headache (12.5%), and infection/sepsis (8.7%). The most common late complications (occurring after 6 weeks of surgery) were endocrinopathy (20.7%), chronic nasal symptoms (2.4%), and cranial nerve palsies (1.9%). They concluded that this meta-analysis demonstrated comparable outcomes between pediatric patients undergoing endoscopic resection of the SBT and the historical figures recorded for open procedures.

Table 1. Skull base pathologies in the case series with >20 children operated via the EAA

	NP	C	PA	RCC	Cho	Oth	GTR	CSF-L	SM	Ex
Locatelli et al., 2010, Pavia and Rome, Italy	27	7 (25.9%)	12 (44.4%)	4 (14.8%)	1 (3.7%)	3 (11.1%)	22 (81.5%)	3 (11.1%)	0	0
Chivukula et al., 2013, Pittsburgh, USA	88	16 (18.1%)	11 (12.5%)	12 (13.6%)	10 (11.3%)	39 (44.3%)	44 (50%)	un***	3** (3.6%)	0
Banu et al., 2014, New York, USA	20	5 (25%)	9 (45%)	0	0	6 (30%)	15 (75%)	0	0	0
Khalili et al., 2015, Pennsylvania, USA	25	13 (52%)	2 (8%)	2 (8%)	2 (8%)	6-(24%)	un	un	un	un
Giovannetti et al., 2018, Rome, Italy	32	12 (37.5%)	8 (25%)	2 (6.2%)	0	10 (31.2%)	un	2 (6.2%)	1** (2.2%)	0
Kim et al., 2019, Seoul, Korea	82	39 (47.5%)	13 (15.8%)	15 (18.2%)	3 (3.6%)	12 (14.6%)	50 (61%)	2 (2.4%)	1* (1.2%)	0
Deopujari et al., 2019, Bombay, India	36	22 (61.1%)	8 (22.2%)	3 (8.3%)	0	3 (8.3%)	un	3 (8.3%)	0	1[1]
Kahilogullari et al., 2019, Ankara, Turkey	41	16 (39%)	12 (29.2%)	0	1 (2.4%)	12 (29.2%)	33 (80.4%)	0	0	1[2]
Total	351	130 (37%)	75 (21.3%)	38 (10.8%)	17 (4.8%)	91 (25.9%)	164 (63.5%)[3]	10 (4.2%)[3]	5 (1.5%)[3]	2 (0.6%)[3]

Cases of angiofibroma, congenital defects, traumatic lesions, and skull base defects, among others were excluded from the analysis (C: Craniopharygioma, Cho: Chordoma, CSF-L: Cerebrospinal fluid leakage, Ex: Exitus, GTR: Gross total resection, NP: Number of patients, Oth: Others, PA: Pituitary adenoma, RCC: Rathke's cleft cyst, SM: Serious morbidity).

*Intraventricular hemorrhage, severe sequelae. **Cerebral abscess. ***unknown in detail.

[1] In a craniopharyngioma case on the postoperative 7th day due to ventriculitis.

[2] In a craniopharyngioma case on the postoperative 15th day due to endocrinological failure and electrolyte imbalance.

[3] unknown series excepted.

As seen in Table 1, we reviewed 8 studies on EEA in children with SBP, which included the series of >20 cases, except for those with angiofibromas, congenital defects, and traumatic and skull base defects. A total of 351 patients were assessed. The most commonly pathology was craniopharygioma (37%; range: 18.1-61.1%). The second-most common pathology was pituitary adenoma (21.3%; range: 8-44.4%), and the third one was RCC (10.8%; range: 0-18.2%). The gross total resection was 63.5% overall (range: 50-81.5%). However, from the series, it can be understood that the success rate was significantly high in the sellar region pathology such as craniopharyngioma, pituitary adenoma, and RCC but not for chordoma and other pathologies in SBP. The overall CSF leakage rate was 4.2% (range: 0-11.1%). Serious morbidity was noted in 1.5% of the patients with intraventricular hemorrhage and cerebral abscess. No patients died during the peri-operative or early postoperative period; however, only 2 patients with craniopharygioma died in the series (0.6%) at 1 and 2 weeks postoperatively due to ventriculitis and deep electrolyte imbalance, respectively.

CONCLUSION

The EEA for SBP is hindered by several difficulties in children, including multiple anatomical challenges, such as variable patterns of pneumatization, narrow piriforme aperture width, and narrow intercarotid distance in the cavernous sinus level [24, 35, 49]. However, despite these difficulties, the EEA in SBP have demonstrated a high success rate with low complication rates in children. One of the disadvantages of this approach is CSF leakage during the surgery with EEA. However, in children, the situation is different. This intervention has shown minimal risk of CSG leakage, especially with the commonly used NF for children all age groups (i.e., from infant to adolescent). The success rate and the preferability of EEA has been consistently increasing with the development of newer technologies and techniques, and this approach is more frequently been applied in children for SBP [44].

PEARLS

SBP are extremely rare in children, and the EEA has gained popularity as an approach for treating these pathologies in children since the years 2000s.

Despite the challenges of small nostril size, narrow corridors, and unpneumatized sphenoid sinus in children, the EEA have been demonstrated to be useful with the use of suitable technological equipment under the guidance of experienced surgeons.

The EEA is a safe and effective approach for SBP not only among adolescents or children but also among infants in suitable cases.

Although the skull base is a meeting point of neurosurgeons and otolaryngologists, it seems that the EEA is developing in the armamentarium of both the units in their consistent efforts and perusal to access the ventral skull base as a team. Our philosophy may be explained with the notion that "four hand," "four eyes," and "two minds" can raise the success rate of this intervention in children. Craniopharyngiomas are most common pathology that is operated via the EEA in children, followed by pituitary adenomas and RCCs. For SBP, in comparison with the other approaches, the EEA has a high success rate and low complication rate, except for postoperative CSF leakage. However, it is believed that the usage of multilayer reconstruction techniques and, especially, with the use of vascularized NF in required cases, the CSF leakage can be significantly decreased by almost the same rates as in other approaches. Over the past 2 decades, the EEA has been increasing preferred and usually the first choice of approach for all types of SBP, especially for sellar pathologies from the frontal sinus to the clivus, in children.

ACKNOWLEDGMENTS

I am grateful to Prof. Cem Meco and Prof Suha Beton as well as all the professors at the Ankara University Department of Otolaryngology who partnered in the endoscopic skull base team and to Prof Agahan Unlu for his mentoring and to my department's professors at the Ankara University, Department of Neurosurgery for their support.

REFERENCES

[1] Azab WA. Pediatric endoscopic endonasal skull base surgery-where do we stand and where we are going? *Childs Nervous System* 35:2079-2080, 2019.

[2] Bakhsheshian J, Jin DL, Chang KE et al. Risk factors associated with the surgical management of craniopharyngiomas in pediatric patients:analysis of 1961 patients from a national registry database. *Neurosurg Focus* 41:E8, 2010.

[3] Banu MA, Guerrero-Maldonado A, McCrea HJ, Garcia-Navarro V, Souweidane MM, Anand VK, Heier L, Schwartz TH, Greenfield JP. Impact of skull base development on endonasal endoscopic surgical corridors. *J Neurosurg Pediatrics* 13:155-169, 2014.

[4] Banu MA, Rathman A, Patel KS, Souweidane MM, Anand VK, Greenfield JP, Schwartz TH. Corridor-based endonasal endoscopic surgery for pediatric skull base pathology with detailed radioanatomic measurements. *Operative Neurosurgery* 10:273-293, 2014.

[5] Basak H, Kahilogullari G, Guler TM, Sayaci YE, Etus V, Meco C. Endonasal endoscopic management of the craniopharyngeal canal meningoencephalocele using a nasoseptal flap in a 6-month-old infant. *Childs Nervous System*, 2020 Nisan. doi: 10.1007/s00381-020-04602-w.

[6] Ben-Ari O, Wengier A, Ringel B, Neiderman NNC, Ram Z, Margalit N, Fliss DM, Abergel A. Nasoseptal flap for skull base reconstruction in children. *J Neurol Surg* B 79:37-41, 2018.

[7] Chen W, Garnder PA, Branstetter BF, Liu SD, Chang YF, Snyderman CH, Goldstein JA, Tyler-Kabara EC, Schuster LA. Long-term impact of pediatric endoscopic endonasal skull base surgery on

midface growth. *J Neurosurg Pediatr* 2019. https://doi.org/10.3171/2018.8.PEDS18183.
[8] Chen G, Zhang Q, Ling F. An endoscopic endonasal approach for the surgical repair of transsphenoidal cephalocele in children. *J Clin Neurosci* 18:723-724, 2011.
[9] Chivukula S, Koutourousiou M, Synderman CH, Fernandez-Miranda JC, Gardner PA, Tyler-Kabara EC. Endoscopic endonasal skull base surgery in the pediatric population. *J Neurosurg Pediatrics* 11:227-241, 2013.
[10] de Divitiis E, Cappabianca P, Gangemi M, Cavallo LM. The role of the endoscopic transsphenoidal approach in pediatric neurosurgery. *Childs Nervous System* 16:692-696, 2000.
[11] Deopujari CE, Shah NJ, Shaikh ST, Karmarkar VS, Mohanty CB. Endonasal endoscopic skull base surgery in children. *Childs Nervous System* 35:2091-2098, 2019.
[12] Di Rocco F, Couloigner V, Dastoli P, Sainte-Rose C, Zerah M, Roger G. Treatment of anterior skull base defects by a transnasal endoscopic approach in children. *J Neurosurg Pediatrics* 6:459-463, 2010.
[13] Duek I, Pener-Tessler A, Yanko-Arzi R, Zaretski A, Abergel A, Safadi A, Fliss DM. Skull base reconstruction in the pediatric patients. *J Neurol Surg* B 79:81-90, 2018.
[14] Elangovan C, Singh PS, Gardner P, Snyderman C, Tyler-Kabara EC, Habeych M, Crammond D, Balzer J, Thirumala PD. Intraoperative neurophysiology monitoring during endoscopic endonasal surgery for pediatric skull base tumors. *J Neurosurg Pediatr* 17:147-155, 2016.
[15] Fliss DM. Recent advances in pediatric skull base surgery. *J Neurol Surg Skull Base* 79:1-2, 2018.
[16] Giovanetti F, Mussa F, Priore P, Scagnet M, Arcovio E, Valentini V, Genitori L. Endoscopic endonasal skull base surgery in pediatric patients. A single center experience. *Journal of Cranio-Maxillo-Facial Surgery* 46:2017-2021, 2018.
[17] Gui S, Zong X, Xinsheng W, Li C, Zhao P, Cao L, Zhang Y. Classification and surgical approaches for transnasal endoscopic

skull base chordoma resection:a 6-year experience with 161 cases. *Neurosurg Rev* 39:321-333, 2016.

[18] Gump WC. Endoscopic endonasal repair of congenital defects of anterior skull base: developmental considerations and surgical outcomes. *J Neurol Surg B Skull Base* 76:291-295, 2015.

[19] Gupta AK, Gupta K, Sunku SK, Modi M, Gupta A. Endoscopic optic nerve fenestration amongst pediatric idiopathic intracranial hypertension: A new surgical option. *Int J Pediatr Otorhinolaryngol* 78:1686-1691, 2014.

[20] Hickman ZL, McDowell MM, Barton SM, Sussman ES, Grunstein E, Anderson RCE. Transnasal endoscopic approach to the pediatric craniovertebral junction and rostral cervical spine: case series and literature review. *Neurosurg Focus* 35:E14, 2013.

[21] Holzmann D, Bozinov O, Krayenbühl N. Is there a place for the endoscope in skull base surgery in children less than 5 years? *J Neurol Surg A Cent Eur Neurosurg* 75:133-139, 2014.

[22] Kahilogullari G, Meco C, Zaimoglu M, Beton S, Meco BC, Tetik B, Unlu A. Pneumocephalus after endoscopic odontoidectomy in a pediatric patient: the lesson learned. *Childs Nervous System* 31(9):1595-1599, 2015.

[23] Kahilogullari G, Yakar F, Bayatlı E, Erden E, Meco C, Unlu A. Endoscopic removal of a suprasellar dermoid cyst in a pediatric patient: a case report and review of the literature. *Childs Nervous System* 34(8):1583-1587, 2018.

[24] Kahilogullari G, Meco C, Beton S, Zaimoglu M, Ozgural O, Basak H, Bozkurt M, Unlu A. Endoscopic transnasal skull base surgery in pediatric patients. *Journal of Neurological Surgery-Part B*, 2019. DOI: https://doi.org/10.1055/s-0039-1692641.

[25] Kassam A, Thomas AJ, Synderman C, Carrau R, Garnder P, Mintz A, Kanaan H, Horowitz M, Pollack IF. Fully endoscopic expanded endonasal approach treating skull base lesions in pediatric patients. *J Neurosurg* (2 Suppl Pediatrics) 106:75-86, 2007.

[26] Keshri AK, Shah SR, Patadia SD, Sahu RN, Behari S. Transnasal endoscopic repair of pediatric meningoencephalocele. *J Pediatr Neurosc* 11:42-45, 2016.

[27] Khalili S, Palmer JN, Adappa ND. The expanded endonasal approach for the treatment of intracranial skull base disease in the pediatric population. *Curr Opin Otolaryngol Head Neck Surg* 23:65-70, 2015.

[28] Kim YH, Lee JY, Phi JH, Wang KC, Kim SK. Endoscopic endonasal skull base surgery for pediatric brain tumors. *Childs Nervous System* 35:2081-2090, 2019.

[29] Kobets A, Ammar A, Dowling K, Cohen A, Goodrich J. The limits of endoscopic endonasal approaches in young children: a review. *Childs Nervous System* 36:263-271, 2020.

[30] Kuan EC, Kaufman AC, Lerner D, Kohanski MA, Tong CCL, Tajudeen BA, Parasher AK, Lee JYK, Storm PB, Palmer JN, Adappa ND. Lack of sphenoid pneumatization does not affect endoscopic endonasal pediatric skull base surgery outcomes. *Laryngoscope* 129:832-836, 2019.

[31] Lee JA, Cooper RL, Nguyen SA, Schlosser RJ, Gudis DA. Endonasal endoscopic surgery for pediatric sellar and suprasellar lesions:a systematic review and meta-analysis. *Otolaryngol Head Neck Surg* Mar 2020 doi:10.1177/0194599820913637.

[32] Locatelli D, Rampa F, Acchiardi I, Bignami M, Pistochini A, Castelnuovo P. Endoscopic endonasal approaches to anterior skull base defects in pediatric patients. *Childs Nervous System* 22:1411-1418, 2006.

[33] Locatelli D, Massimi L, Rigante M, Custodi V, Paludetti G, Castelnuova P, Di Rocco C. Endoscopic endonasal transsphenoidal surgery for sellar tumors in children. *Int J Pediatr Otorhinolaryngol* 74:1298-1302, 2010.

[34] Locatelli D, Veiceschi P, Castelnuovo P, Tanriover N, Evliyaoglu O, Canaz H, Ugurlar D, Gazioglu N. Transsphenoidal surgery for pituitary adenomas in pediatric patients:a multicentric retrospective study. *Childs Nervous System* 35:2119-2126, 2019.

[35] London NR, Rangel GG, Walz PC. The expanded endonasal approach in pediatric skull base surgery: A review. *Laryngoscope Investigate Otolaryngology* 5:313-325, 2020.

[36] Ma J, Huang Q, Li X, Huang D, Xian J, Cui S, Li Y, Zhou B. Endoscopic transnasal repair of cerebrospinal fluid leaks with and without an encephalocele in pediatric patients: from infant to children. *Childs Nervous System* 31:1493-1498, 2015.

[37] Madhok R, Prevedello D, Gardner P, Carrau R, Snyderman CH, Kassam AB. Endoscopic endonasal resection of Rathke cleft cyst:clinical outcomes and surgical nuances. *J Neurosurg* 112:1333-1339, 2010.

[38] Massimi L, Rigante M, D'Angelo L, Paternoster G, Leonardi P, Paludetti G, Di Rocco C. Quality of postoperative course in children:endoscopic endonasal surgery versus sublabial microsurgery. *Acta Neurochir* 153:843-849, 2011.

[39] Nation J, Schupper AJ, Deconde A, Levy M. Pediatric endoscopic endonasal approaches for skull base lesions in the very young: Is it safe and effective? *J Neurol Surg B* 79:574-579, 2018.

[40] Nation J, Schupper AJ, Deconde A, Levy M. CSF leak after endoscopic skull base surgery in children: A single institution experience. *International Journal of Pediatric Otorhinolaryngology* 119:22-26, 2019.

[41] Ozgural O, Kahilogullari G, Dogan I, Al-Beyati ESM, Bozkurt M, Tetik B, Comert A, Meco C, Unlu A. Single-center surgical experience of the treatment of craniopharyngiomas with emphasis on the operative approach: endoscopic endonasal and open microscopic transcranial approaches. *J Craniofac Surg* 29(6):e572-e578, 2018.

[42] Parasher A, Lerner DK, Glicksman JT, Storm PB, Lee JYK, Vossough A, Brooks S, Palmer JN, Adappa ND. The impact of expanded endonasal skull base surgery on midfacial growth in pediatric patients. *Laryngoscope*, 130:338-342, 2020.

[43] Patel S, Thamboo A, Quon J et al. Outcomes after andoscopic endonasal resection of craniopharyngiomas in the pediatric population. *World Neurosurgery* 108:6-14, 2017.

[44] Rastatter JC, Snyderman CH, Gardner PA, Alden TD, Tyler-Kabara E. Endoscopic endonasal surgery for sinonasal and skull base lesions in the pediatric population. *Otolaryngol Clin N Am* 48:79-99, 2015.
[45] Rigante M, Massimi L, Parrilla C, Galli J, Calderelli M, Di Rocco C, Paludetti G. Endoscopic transsphenoidal approach versus microscopic approach in children. *International Journal of Pediatric Otorhinolaryngology* 75:1132-1136, 2011.
[46] Shah RN, Surowitz JB, Patel MR, Huang BY, Snyderman CH, Carrau RL, Kassam AB, Germanwala AV, Zanation AM. Endoscopic pedicled nasoseptal flap reconstruction for pediatric skull base defects. *Laryngoscope* 119:1067-1075, 2009.
[47] Shenouda K, Yuhan BT, Mir A, Gonik N, Eloy JA, Liu JK, Folbe AJ, Svider PF. Endoscopic resection of pediatric skull base tumors:an evidence-based review. *J Neurol Surg B* 80:527-539, 2019.
[48] Shepard MJ, Elzoghby MA, Kiehna EN, Payne SC, Jane JA. Presentation and outcomes in surgically and conservatively managed pediatric Rathe cleft cysts. *J Neurosurg Pediatr* 21:308-314, 2018.
[49] Singh H, Greenfield JP, Anand VK, Schwartz TH. *Pediatric endonasal endoscopic skull base surgery: A case-based manual.* EndoPress. 1st edition, Tuttlingen, Germany, pp: 1-34, 2016.
[50] Stapleton AL, Tyler-Kabara EC, Gardner PA, Snyderman CH, Wang EW. Risk factors for cerebrospinal fluid leak in pediatric patients undergoing endoscopic endonasal skull base surgery. *International Journal of Otorhinolaryngology* 93:163-166, 2017.
[51] Tan SH, Ganesan D, Prepageran N, Waran V. A minimally invasive endoscopic transnasal approach to the craniovertebral junction in the pediatric population. *Eur Arch Otorhinolaryngol* 271:3101-3105, 2014.
[52] Tatreau JR, Patel MR, Shah R, McKinney KA, Wheless SA, Senior BA, Ewend MG, Germanwala AV, Ebert CS, Zanation AM. Anatomical consideratins for endoscopic endonasal skull base surgery in pediatric patients. *Laryngoscope* 120:1730-1737, 2010.

[53] Yakar F, Dogan I, Meco C, Heper AO, Kahilogullari G. Sellar embryonal tumor: a case report and review of the literature. *Asian J Neurosurg* 13(4):1197-1201, 2008.

[54] Youssef CA, Smortherman CR, Kraemer DF, Aldana RP. Predicting the limits of the endoscopic endonasal approach in children: a radiological anatomical study. *J Neurosurg Pediatr* 17:510-515, 2016.

[55] Zhan R, Xin T, Li X, Li W, Li X. Endonasal endoscopic transsphenoidal approach to lesions of the seller region in pediatric patients. *The Journal of Craniofacial Surgery* 26:1818-1822, 2015.

[56] Zoli M, Milanese L, Bonfatti R, Faustini-Fustuni M, Marucci G, Tallini G, Zenesini C, Sturiale C, Frank G, Pasquini E, Mazzatenta D. Clival chordomas:considerations after 16 years of endoscopic endonasal surgery. *J Neurosurg* 128:329-338, 2018.

Chapter 5

ENDOSCOPE–ASSISTED MICROSURGERY OF PEDIATRIC BRAIN TUMORS

Mohamed A. El Beltagy[1,2,*], *MD, PhD* and *Mostafa M. E. Atteya, MD*

[1]Children's Cancer Hospital Egypt (CCHE), Cairo, Egypt
[2]Kasr Al Ainy School of Medicine, Cairo University, Cairo, Egypt

ABSTRACT

Endoscope-assisted microsurgery (EAMS) refers to the addition of neuroendoscopy as an adjunct to ordinary open microsurgical techniques to enable closer inspection of the hidden corners of the operative field and to increase the chances of achieving better extents of safe tumor resections through augmenting their benefits and obviating the drawbacks of both techniques by simultaneous or tandem integration. This chapter sheds lights on the potential benefits of EAMS in the management of complex pediatric brain tumors in the most crucial areas of the brain and the skull base through the main major neurosurgical approaches. Technical details and precautions are also covered, giving particular attention to patient safety and complication avoidance. A special focus is

---

* Corresponding Author's E-mail: beltagy_mohamed@hotmail.com.

directed towards handling techniques, intraoperative decision making, operative steps, chronological staging, role of the assisting surgeon, and harmony within the surgical team. EAMS is especially helpful in tumors occupying the suprasellar region, cerebello-pontine angles, and the ventricular system. There is a definitive learning curve for EAMS which could be achieved by keen practicing especially in large supratentorial intra-parenchymal surgical cavities where training on these techniques could be safer.

INTRODUCTION

The earliest reports of endoscopic neurosurgery go back to the early 20th century. L'Espinasse and Doyen reported early endoscopic surgery for the choroid plexus and the posterior fossa [1-4]. An era of advancement in the technology and the industry of endoscopes progressed in the 1980s [5] during which microscopic neurosurgical techniques were dominating at that time with their superior panoramic views and 3-D images.

The technical advancements in the optics of endoscopes together with the invention of suitable microsurgical instruments paved the way to the introduction of the endoscope to complement the microscope in the same surgical procedure; thus, giving the surgeon unprecedented flexibility to look around the hidden surgical corners and to view the morbid neurovascular anatomy in close, highly illuminated, and angled views unobtainable by the straight optics of the surgical microscope.

This chapter will discuss the potential benefits of endoscope-assisted microsurgery (EAMS) in different pediatric brain tumors. More light will be shed upon craniopharyngioma surgery and cerebello-pontine angle tumors being the two entities which benefit much from EAMS. Technical tricks, pitfalls, and different tactics in EAMS will be mentioned accordingly.

CRANIOPHARYNGIOMA SURGERY

Craniopharyngioma surgery is considered one of the most difficult skull base surgeries. It is challenging in terms of the eloquent nature of the morbid neuroanatomy related and the critical possible attachments of the tumor to the optic pathways, the hypothalamus, internal carotid artery, and the pituitary gland. In the mind of surgeon, there should be always a logical balance between the extent of resection and the function left for the child to live with. Not only does this depend on the preoperative imaging, but also it depends on the intraoperative findings and the dissectability of the tumor from the hypothalamus and the surrounding critical neurovascular structures.

Microscopic surgery has been considered the gold standard for craniopharyngioma surgery for decades [6, 7]. However, the new developments in the optics and neuroendoscopy have reserved a good place for endoscopic maneuvers to help in achieving better operative and functional outcomes in those critical surgeries.

Craniopharyngioma surgery is usually time consuming. That is why the surgeon might be exhausted when he is approaching the final stages of surgery. That may result in overlooking residual tumors and reluctancy in using the endoscope to have the final look to avoid leaving tumors behind. The endoscope was found to be extremely helpful in the assessment of the hidden corners of the operative field and the undersurface of the visual pathways where the microscope cannot easily because the operative microscope functions only in straight optical lines (Figure 1).

The consistency of the tumor, the size, and the local invasiveness and attachability to the surroundings affect the timing and the technique of endoscopic assistance. If the tumor is quite small, it may leave enough room for the endoscope to operate. The possible corridors for endoscopic introduction are the carotid oculomotor triangle, the optical carotid triangle, the Inter optic space, and the lamina terminalis. However, if the tumor is large enough and contains significant solid parts that exert pressure on the surrounding potential anatomic spaces, the introduction of endoscope will be more feasible only after debulking some parts of the solid tumor and creating room to allow safe endoscopic assistance. Continuous irrigation is mandatory to avoid thermal injury to these intricate neurovascular structures.

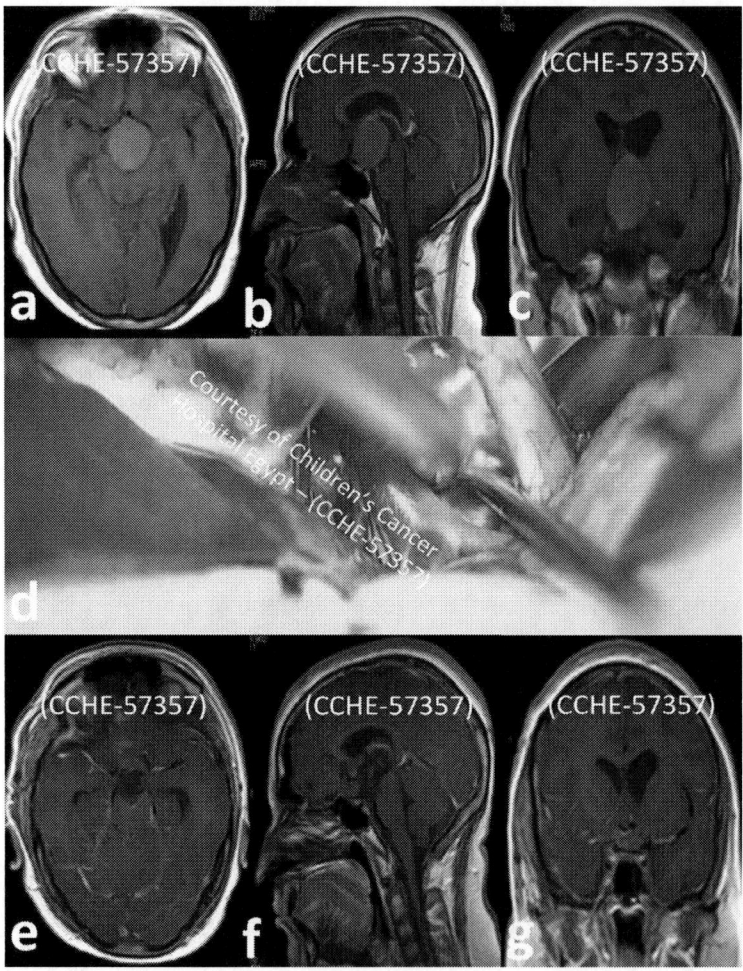

Figure 1. EAMS of craniopharyngiomas, two instruments' variation. a-c: pre-operative contrast enhanced MRI showing a large craniopharyngioma with hypothalamic extension. Endoscopic assistance enabled revealed that the tumor was dissectible from the hypothalamus which enabled total safe excision of the tumor. d: a microscopic left pterional view showing the endoscopic shaft that is held by the assistant and is introduced through the inter-optic window. The surgeon is working through the optic-carotid triangle with two instruments. e-g: early post-operative MRI showing total tumor excision [Courtesy of Children's Cancer Hospital Egypt (CCHE-57357)].

It is important to note that the angled lenses may be used to assess hidden corners such as under the optic chiasm and the Liliequist membrane. The tip of the endoscope is not seen on the endoscopic monitor. So, it is the assistant's rule to closely monitor the location of the endoscopic tip in order to avoid neurovascular injuries.

It is also crucial to mention that the endoscope-assisted surgery of craniopharyngioma should only be performed by experienced neurosurgeons and assistants due to the narrow anatomical windows available in between the critical neurovascular structures and to avoid disastrous injuries. There is a definite learning curve for endoscope-assisted microsurgery. A good advice for the beginners is to practice these maneuvers first in large open supratentorial surgical cavities to gradually gain cumulative experience and acquire the operative sensitivity of handling the endoscope both in dynamic and static fashions.

SURGERY OF THE LATERAL VENTRICULAR TUMORS

Lateral ventricular tumors are not infrequent in the pediatric age group and usually these tumors reach large sizes before diagnosis [8, 9]. Sometimes, the neurosurgeon faces a hemispheric brain tumor; and this is quite a challenge in children because of the narrow limits of blood loss, operative time, and the delicacy of their brains. So, meticulous hemostasis and delicate maneuvers are the cornerstones of surgery of large ventricular tumors in those children.

A good technique we utilize is the transcortical introduction of the endoscope. After craniotomy has been performed, the endoscope is introduced transcortically guided by the neuro-navigation. This allows early identification of the tumor's vascular pedicle (Figures 2 and 3) and gives an opportunity for early proper hemostasis and significantly makes further surgery easier. This is especially useful in children harboring large choroid plexus papillomas and meningiomas. Once the tumor's vascular pedicle is coagulated through the early transcortical endoscope, the rest of surgery usually becomes smooth, without much bleeding, and the consistency of the tumors usually becomes softer after devascularization.

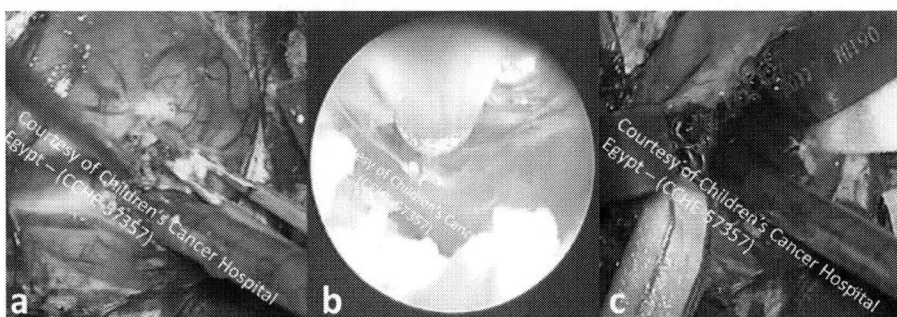

Figure 2. Early control of tumor's vascular pedicle via EAMS of lateral ventricular tumors. a. early transcortical introduction of the endoscope after craniotomy to directly inspect the tumor, its boundaries, the degree of vascularity, and trying to identify the tumor's vascular pedicle for early control. b. endoscopic-assisted coagulation of the tumor's vascular pedicle. c. completion of the approach with the microscope under direct endoscopic guidance to the coagulated tumor pedicle and the discovered cleavage planes [Courtesy of Children's Cancer Hospital Egypt (CCHE-57357)].

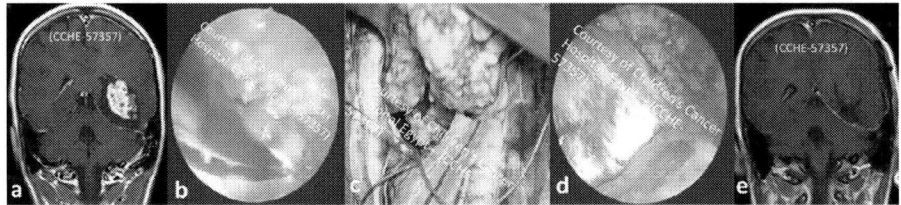

Figure 3. EAMS of an intraventricular meningioma. a: Preoperative contrast enhanced T1 coronal MRI showing left occipital horn tumor. b: creation of a cleavage plane under the endoscopic assistance with microscissors. c: excision of the de-vascularized tumor under the surgical microscope. d: surgical bed after gross total excision. e: early post-operative contrast-enhanced coronal MRI showing total excision of the tumor [Courtesy of Children's Cancer Hospital Egypt (CCHE-57357)].

The endoscope allows the surgeon to achieve flexible trajectory changes and to get different angles of vision which allow closer inspection of the boundaries is of these large tumors and creating nice tumor cleavage planes within the ventricular spaces which are already narrowed by the mass effect of these large tumors. Neuronavigation and intraoperative ultrasonography are very helpful adjuncts during surgical excisions of these challenging intraventricular tumors.

SURGERY OF CEREBELLO-PONTINE ANGLE (CPA) TUMORS

The cerebello-pontine angle is considered one of the most complex regions in the central nervous system. It is a narrow space that is crowded with the lower cranial nerves, the brainstem, the cerebellum, and the major vessels of the posterior circulation. Tumor excision is a real challenge when it comes to this intricate location. The most common tumors that arise in this critical region are vestibular schwannomas, meningiomas, and epidermoid cysts.

Vestibular schwannomas are known to displace the facial nerve anteriorly in most cases and superiorly in fewer cases. Moreover, tumoral invasion inside the internal auditory canal adds significant challenge to these surgeries. Endoscopic assistance in vestibular schwannoma surgery enables early identification of the facial nerve and thus provides early protection of this nerve. Also, this technique allows identification of tumors inside the internal auditory canal before opening the canal and without exerting any retraction. Using the endoscope early in the procedure allows the surgeon to minimize cerebellar retraction and enables the release of cerebral spinal fluid (CSF) and thus achieving more and more relaxation of the surgical bed without retracting the cerebellum significantly. Also, endoscopic assessment facilitates the detection of open air cells and confirms sealing them properly, and this diminishes the incidence of postoperative CSF leaks.

It has to be mentioned that due to the narrow spaces in the CPA, and the crowdedness of the neurovascular structures, using the endoscope in this critical region should only be practiced by highly experienced surgeons to avoid neurovascular injuries.

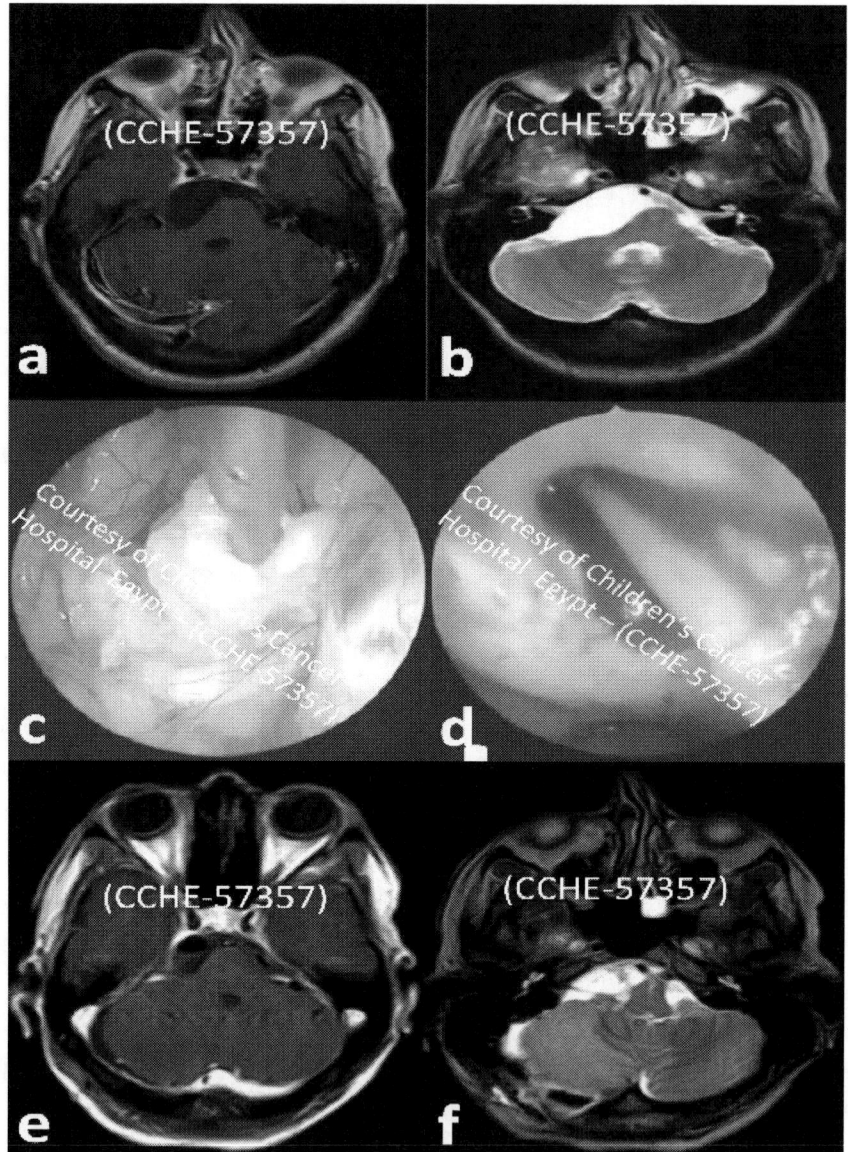

Figure 4. EAMS of a right CPA epidermoid tumor. a-b: pre-operative MRI. c. early endoscopic guided assistance in piece-meal tumor excision in between the cranial nerves in the CPA. The tumor exhibits the characteristic pearly white texture.
d. endoscopic inspection of the interior of the lateral part of the internal auditory canal; a unique view that is not obtainable by the microscope. g-i: early post-operative MRI showing total tumor excision [Courtesy of Children's Cancer Hospital Egypt (CCHE-57357)].

The epidermoid tumors are known for insinuating themselves in between the cranial nerves and extending into hidden corners and potential anatomical spaces. The use of endoscopic assistance in CPA tumors is helpful specially in the assessment of the hidden corners of the operative field and undersurface of the cranial nerves and the lateral surface of the IAC using zero, 30-, 45-, and 70-degrees endoscopic lenses accordingly. When using angled endoscopic lenses, extra caution must be exerted to observe the tip of the endoscope which is not readily seen on the monitor and here comes the task of the assistant surgeon to be completely devoted to this point during the dynamic movements of the endoscope inside the CPA keeping in mind that the endoscope movement is both rotatory and linear with angled lenses, and that the direction of endoscopic handling is not the same as of the visual input received on the endoscopic monitor. It goes without saying that intraoperative neurophysiological monitoring and neuronavigation are very important adjuncts in these CPA surgeries. Figure 4 shows endoscope-assisted excision of a CPA epidermoid cyst.

SURGERY OF FOURTH VENTRICULAR TUMORS

The most common tumors which invade the fourth ventricle in children are astrocytoma, ependymoma, medulloblastoma, and brain stem gliomas [10]. The application of the endoscopic assisted microsurgery of fourth ventricular tumor is helpful for the close assessment of the boundaries, attachments, and adhesions to the surrounding structures.

Once debulking is started, the endoscope or pediscope can be introduced, and the breakdown of adhesions could be carried out under endoscopic view to release the tumor from the lateral recesses of the fourth ventricle and the vermis of the cerebellum and to closely inspect any adhesions or invasion of the brainstem at an early stage of the surgery with minimal or no cerebellar retraction.

This enables the surgeon to circumferentially release the tumor from the surroundings and to appreciate any brain stem invasion ahead without exertion of any traction on the brain stem or cerebellar tissues. The minimized retraction results in less postoperative edema and potentially in a better functional outcome especially in terms of the cerebellar mutism spectrum. Figure 5 shows endoscope-assisted creation of tumor cleavage planes and breakdown of adhesions in the lateral recesses of the fourth ventricle.

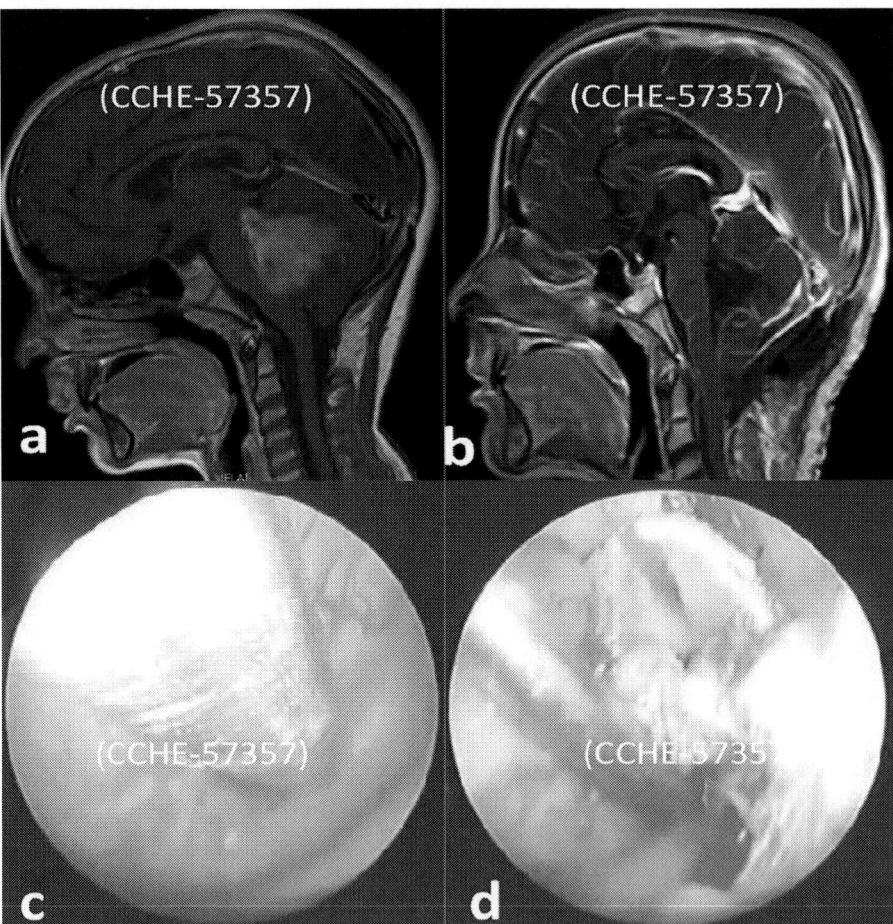

Figure 5. EAMS of a fourth ventricular medulloblastoma. a. pre-operative contrast-enhanced sagittal MRI showing a large fourth ventricular enhancing tumor reaching the pineal region. b. post-operative contrasted enhanced sagittal MRI showing total tumor excision. c. endoscope-assisted dissection of the lateral recess and creating cleavage planes. d. breakdown of the adhesions between the tumor and neural tissues by sharp scissors [Courtesy of Children's Cancer Hospital Egypt (CCHE-57357)].

SURGICAL FOR PARENCHYMAL TUMORS OF THE CEREBRUM, CEREBELLUM, AND THE BRAIN STEM

Due to the straight optical lines of the microscope, some remnant tumors could be missed in the corners of the resection cavity, and it usually requires some retraction to look around the boundaries of the surgical cavity. Moreover, the funnel or the flask shaped surgical cavity increases the opportunity of leaving a hidden tumor residual. The endoscopic assistance in this situation is helpful in detecting any residual tumors without significant retraction.

In lesions such as arteriovenous malformations, cavernomas, and highly vascular brain tumors, endoscopic assistance is valuable in preventing postoperative surgical bed hematomas. As mentioned before, a tedious learning curve is required before mastering these endoscopic assisted techniques, and therefore, practicing EAMS during the excision of large parenchymal tumors could be a good opportunity to improve the learning curve and master the techniques and the handling of endoscope during these types of surgeries with a relatively safer endoscopic navigation.

OPERATIVE ROOM SETUP AND IMAGE INTEGRATION

Proper setup of the operative room and the equipment setting is mandatory for the success of the EAMS and for saving time during procedure and anesthesia. Different forms of image integration have been proposed. Whatever the technique of endoscopic optical output or integration adopted, the location of the devices and monitors should be designed to minimize the efforts exerted by the surgeon, assistant and the nurses to follow the different optical outputs and the operative procedures performed. The ideal setup allows the whole team to watch output monitors with eye movements rather than cervical spine or body movements.

OPERATIVE STEPS OF EAMS AND THEIR CHRONOLOGICAL STAGING

There are three groups of situations during which the endoscope could be introduced to achieve an added benefit. In other words, there are three scenarios to the possible timing of endoscopic use in each procedure to assist the operative microscope: first, the earliest initial endoscopic assessment of the surgical bed, boundaries, and attachments. This "look around" scenario is only possible if there is enough room in both the surgical corridor and the operative bed. This room could be found in some circumstances with little manipulation and in other circumstances it could be only created after some debulking and dissection maneuvers. In large tumors and tight spaces however, the endoscope may not be possibly introducible until significant part of the surgery has been carried out first by the microscope to create some room for endoscopic assistance.

Second, the endoscope is introduce in the intermediate section of surgery either to achieve a planned purpose such as examination of the tumoral invasion of the IAC, undersurface of certain cranial nerves and the dissectability of certain tumor parts, or simply to check the whole field and the hidden corners that are difficult or impossible to assess using the straight microscopic optical lines; and this step can be repeated "on-demand" many times in alternation or combination with the microscope. The time spent on these techniques could be markedly diminished by proper preoperative room setup and correct equipment setting as mentioned above.

The last phase is the final check on the extent of resection and the resectability of tumor residual attached to critical structures such as the hypothalamus, pituitary stalk, and cranial nerves to decide whether to elect to trials at total excision versus leaving minor residual to ensure safety and functionality. This endoscope-based decision making was found very helpful in large craniopharyngiomas to determine whether the residual is dissectible and to guide the safest extent of resection.

SURGICAL HARMONY AND ENDOSCOPIC HANDLING FOR EAMS

The success of EAMS depends greatly on the harmony and the mutual understanding between the surgeon and the assistant and the steadiness of their procedures. Any moment of lack of concentration or unintended movement within the surgical field could result in a significant morbidity to the patient. The assistant's eyes work during EAMS in a "nystagmoid fashion" to bounce repeatedly between the endoscopic monitor and the microscopic or the naked-eye input of the surgical field. This is especially important if the endoscopic lens used for wandering is not of a zero degree because the direction of movement of the shaft of endoscope will not be exactly the same as of the movement perceived on the monitor.

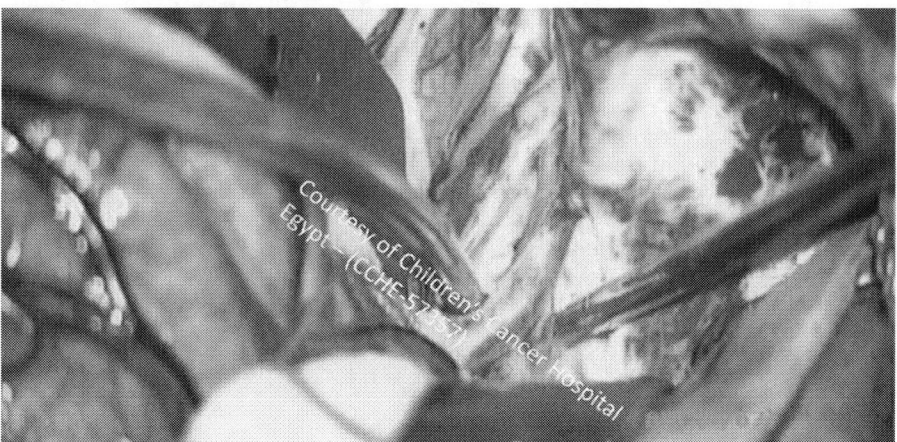

Figure 6. A single instrument variation of EAMS. The surgeon is introducing the endoscope with one hand through the carotid-oculomotor triangle; and is manipulating tissues with the suction tip held in the other hand through the carotid-optic window [Courtesy of Children's Cancer Hospital Egypt (CCHE-57357)].

There are three common handling tactics for EAMS that are utilized interchangeably according to the operative circumstances and the purpose intended. First, the assistant holds the endoscope in a dynamic fashion in harmony with the surgeon's tissue manipulations. There should be mutual arrangement of the best space utilization within the surgical corridor and deep within the operative bed. This understanding subsequently controls the number and type of instruments to be used and the range of motion allowed in every moment accordingly. Usually, both surgeon's hands are free to work with two instruments such as a suction tube and a microdissector and the endoscope is held dynamically by the assistant (Figure 1).

Second, the well-trained surgeon can handle the endoscope by one hand and work around the neural elements with a single instrument in his other hand in harmony with the assistant. This method is helpful during the "look around" phase of EAMS which is essentially an observant phase during which not much tissue manipulation is required, so, a single instrument in the surgeon's hand does the job (Figure 6).

Third, the endoscope is attached to a rigid fixator attached to the operating table. This tactic is however considered the most critical among the tactics described here because extra care should be exercised to prevent inadvertent movements to the fixing arm or the operating table. The surgeon and the assistant hands are free and can cooperate at this step utilizing various microsurgical instruments. The assistant, however, can use one of his hands to ensure stability and security of the endoscope and its holding arm during this phase.

CONCLUSION

Endoscopic assisted microsurgical techniques of pediatric brain tumors provide high resolution images of the operative field and the relevant critical neurovascular structures and hidden surgical corners under bright illumination with the ability to look around with varying sets of lenses in regions inaccessible by the straight optics of the microscope and without retraction or tissue trauma. This is helpful in pediatric tumors in the sella, CPA, ventricles, and supratentorial or infratentorial parenchymal tumors. In EAMS, the endoscope complements the surgical microscope with the above-mentioned merits and in return the microscope provides a wide panoramic 3-D environment to control most of the procedure in alternation or combination with the endoscope. There is a gradual learning curve in EAMS, and these techniques should be performed by experienced surgeons. Parenchymal tumors with large resection cavities are good opportunities for practicing EAMS.

REFERENCES

[1] Dandy, W. (1922). An operative procedure for hydrocephalus. *Johns Hopkins Hosp. Bull.* 33:189–190.

[2] Doyen, E. (1917). *Surgical therapeutics and operative techniques*, vol 1. (Bailliere/Tindall and Cox, London, 599–602).

[3] Gieger, M., Cohen, A. (1995). "The history of neuroendoscopy." In: *Minimally invasive techniques in neurosurgery*, edited by Cohen, A. and Haines, S., 1-5. (Williams & Wilkins, Baltimore 1995).

[4] Cohen, A. (1996). Endoscopic neurosurgery. In: "*Neurosurgery.*" Edited by Wilkins, R. and Rengachary. S., 539–546. McGraw Hill. (New York 1996).

[5] Epstein, M. (1980). Endoscopy: developments in optical instrumentation. *Science.* 210(4467):280-5. doi: 10.1126/science. 7423188.

[6] Laws, E. R. Jr. (1980). Transsphenoidal microsurgery in the management of craniopharyngioma. *J. Neurosurg.* 52(5):661-666. doi: 10.3171/jns.1980.52.5.0661.

[7] Symon, L. (1983). Microsurgery of the hypothalamus with special reference to craniopharyngioma. *Neurosurg. Rev.* 6(2):43-49 doi: 10.1007/BF01743032.

[8] Elwatidy, S. M., Albakr, A. A., Al Towim, A. A., Malik, S. H. (2017). Tumors of the lateral and third ventricle: surgical management and outcome analysis in 42 cases. *Neurosciences (Riyadh).* 22(4):274-281. doi: 10.17712/nsj.2017.4.20170149.

[9] Zuccaro, G., Sosa, F., Cuccia, V., Lubieniecky, F., Monges, J. (1999). Lateral ventricle tumors in children: a series of 54 cases. *Childs Nerv. Syst.* 15(11-12):774-785. doi: 10.1007/s003810050470.

[10] Riaz, Q., Naeem, E., Fadoo, Z., Lohano, M., Mushtaq, N. (2019). Intracranial tumors in children: a 10-year review from a single tertiary health-care center. *Childs Nerv. Syst.* 35(12):2347-2353. doi: 10.1007/ s00381-019-04260-7. Epub 2019 Jul 2. PMID: 31267185.

In: Neuroendoscopic Procedures ... ISBN: 978-1-68507-092-2
Editor: Soner Duru   © 2021 Nova Science Publishers, Inc.

Chapter 6

SUPRASELLAR ARACHNOID CYSTS: RETROSPECTIVE SERIES AND LITERATURE REVIEW

E. Marcati[*], *MD, G. L. Gribaudi*[†], *MD, M. Cenzato*[‡], *MD and G. Talamonti*[§], *MD*
Department of Neurosurgery, ASST Niguarda Hospital, Milan, Italy

ABSTRACT

Suprasellar arachnoid cysts (SACs) are benign collections of cerebrospinal fluid (CSF). They are reported to amount to around 9-11% of all intracranial arachnoid cysts. Wide literature exists on their origin and pathogenesis where the majority of the authors described them as congenital lesions, due to a diverticular expansion of an abnormal membrane of Liliequist or interpeduncular cistern, which cause a partial or complete obstruction of CSF.

---

[*] Corresponding Author's E-mail: eleonora.marcati@ospedaleniguarda.it.
[†] Corresponding Author's E-mail: giulialetizia.gribaudi@ospedaleniguarda.it.
[‡] Corresponding Author's E-mail: marco.cenzato@ospedaleniguarda.it.
[§] Corresponding Author's E-mail: giuseppe.talamonti@ospedaleniguarda.it.

Typically, SACs expand from the prepontine space, displacing and blocking the third ventricle and/or the aqueduct, finally causing obstructive hydrocephalus. Most of the arachnoid cysts are asymptomatic and recognized incidentally with increasing frequency since the introduction of MR imaging. Presence of clinical signs or symptoms represents the main surgical indication. The treatment of these cysts is surgical.

Endoscopic surgery has been advocated as the primary treatment for SACs with hydrocephalus, superior to large craniotomy or shunting. Moreover, ventriculocystocisternotomy has been found to have a higher success rate than ventriculocystostomy. Instead, the choice of the best treatment is still unclear for SACs without associated hydrocephalus.

The main classification system which divides these cysts in communicating (upper diverticulum of the diencephalic membrane, from the prepontine cistern) or non-communicating (cystic dilatation of the interpeduncular cistern) has been recently reviewed by André et al. adding the asymmetrical type 3, which expands to other subarachnoid spaces.

We report here our series of 18 patients with SACs who were treated at our Department in a 15-year period. We describe the endoscopic approach and analyse the clinical and radiological follow-up. The mean follow-up was 80 months.

There were no mortality and no permanent morbidity. Patients with a type 3 cyst (5.5%) required a ventriculoperitoneal shunt because of persistent hydrocephalus. The majority of patients (94.5%) clinically improved except for one who remained unchanged throughout the follow-up. Radiological results were excellent in all cases.

This chapter aims to underline the importance of anatomical and pathophysiological aspects and classification systems to choose the best surgical approach for each different subtype. Adding our experience, we agreed with other authors that there is a limited role for open surgery and we recognize as well that the gold standard for SACs is nowadays the dual endoscopic fenestration.

INTRODUCTION

Arachnoid cysts (ACs) are benign intracranial collections of cerebrospinal fluid (CSF) lined out with arachnoid membranes. They are found to occur more often in males than females, by a ratio of nearly 2:1 and account for 1-2% of all intracranial space-occupying lesions (Albuquerque and Giannotta, 1997; Mustansir et al., 2018). ACs are most often diagnosed in childhood (almost 60-90% of all arachnoid cysts), at a mean age of 6 years with a significant peak (85%) in incidence before age 2 (Gui et al., 2011). In rare cases, they can be detected antenatally in routine ultrasound (US) exams and magnetic resonance imaging (MRI) (McCrea et al., 2015, Talamonti et al., 2011). More than 75% of arachnoid cysts arise in the supratentorial compartment; approximately 9 to 15% occur in the sellar and suprasellar areas (Invergo et al., 2012; Rengachary and Watanabe, 1981). André et al. reported the incidence of suprasellar cysts up to 21% of all pediatric arachnoid cysts related to the improvement in diagnostic tools, especially MRI (André et al., 2016).

The arachnoid membrane develops at 2-3 months of gestational age (GA) and suprasellar arachnoid cysts (SACs) are described usually later than other localizations, around the third trimester, as a diverticulum of Liliequist's membrane (Crimmins et al., 2006). Their presence in utero and their high prevalence in children with no history of trauma support the hypothesis of a congenital origin (Gui et al., 2011). Conversely, Al-Holou et al. reported an increasing prevalence peak from 3.8% at 1 to 4.6% at 5 years of age, suggesting a postnatal development (Invergo et al., 2012; Al-Holou et al., 2010; Juan et al., 2011).

Although the majority of SACs have been described to be stable in the long term (Schachenmayr and Friede, 1979; Invergo et al., 2012), our group according to Al-Holou et al. reported patients younger than 4 years of age at presentation having a cyst enlargement (Al- Holou et al., 2010; Talamonti et al., 2011).

Several reports described associated malformations such as agenesis of the corpus callosum, midline septi, and tonsillar descent.

In 1935 Barlow reported the first case of a suprasellar arachnoid cyst. A 29-years-old man complaining of retrobulbar pain and headache, especially marked on sneezing or coughing, showed a "cystic tumor" coming from the pituitary fossa beneath the chiasm, which was found to arise from the subchiasmal arachnoid membrane (Barlow, 1935).

ETIOPATHOGENESIS

The first case of arachnoid cyst was described by Bright in 1831, who attributed the pathogenesis to an anomalous splitting of the arachnoid membrane, a theory later confirmed by Starkman et al. and Krawchenko et al., regarding SACs (Adeeb et al., 2013; Bright, 1831; Starkman et al., 1958; Krawchenko et al., 1979).

Kasdon et al. in 1977, as well as Fox and Al Mefty in 1980, described SACs as divertula or outpouchings of the Liliequist's membrane made imperforate by previous haemorrhage, infection, or maldevelopment, which begins as a Liliequist diverticulum and expands until, in some cases, the caudal opening seals off, leaving an enclosed cyst. Consequently, at the level of the suprasellar cistern, a partial or complete obstruction of CSF flow can be found (Kasdon et al., 1977; Binitie et al., 1984; Santamarta et al., 1995; Fox and Al-Mefty, 1980).

Therefore, primary congenital cysts arise from the splitting of the arachnoid membrane in utero, while secondary cysts, far less common, are secondary to trauma, surgery, intracranial haemorrhage or infection (Lewis, 1962; Invergo et al., 2012).

"Active fluid secretion" and "pulsatile pump" mechanisms are the two main actual primary cysts theories.

Active Fluid Secretion Theory

Microvilli with secreting and absorptive properties, ATPase, and alkaline phosphatase have been found on the inner surface of the cysts sustaining the idea of an active fluid mechanism involved in the origin and expansion of the cyst. When the secretion fails to be drained by dural sinus is collected by the microvilli in a closed cyst (Santamarta et al., 1995; Go et al., 1984).

Furthermore, Sandberg et al. found a higher protein concentration of cyst content compared to CSF in 34% of the cases (Sandberg et al., 2005).

Pulsatile Mechanism Pump (Ball Valve Hypothesis) Theory

Williams and Guthkelch, in 1974, suggested that a communication between the subarachnoid space and the cyst could act as a oneway valve and the enlargement of arachnoid cysts could be related to a 'pulsatile pump mechanism' (Williams et al., 1974). Santamarta et al. described a slit of the arachnoid attached to the basilar artery, where it pierces the basal leaf of Liliequist's membrane, and considered the arterial inflow responsible for the pressure gradient between the subarachnoid space and the cyst (Santamarta et al., 1995; Schroeder and Gaab, 1997).

Conversely, Williams et al. and Du Boulay et al. considered the arterial inflow to be inefficient and emphasised the responsiveness to venous pressure gradients, during Valsalva manoeuvers (Williams et al., 1974; Du Boulay, 1966; Du Boulay et al., 1972).

The content of arachnoid cysts resembles more that of CSF, supporting this latter theory as confirmed in endoscopic studies, especially when considering suprasellar cysts and their relationship to the basilar artery and Liliequist's membrane.

CLASSIFICATION

To better understand suprasellar cysts, the anatomy of Liliequist's membranes has to be briefly reviewed. Liliequist's membrane is composed of two arachnoid sheets, the diencephalic and the mesencephalic membranes.

The diencephalic leaf arises from the dorsum sellae and the posterior clinoid process going upward and backward, attaching to the pia mater of the inferior surface or the diencephalon between the infundibulum and the mammillary bodies.

The mesencephalic leaf arises from the dorsum sellae and goes downward, but is not directly attached to the brain posteriorly. It can extend to the outer arachnoid membranes that surround the basilar artery in the prepontine space, which is the inferior wall of the interpeduncular cistern, separated from the prepontine cistern (André et al., 2016; Froelich et al., 2008).

A first classification of SACs was proposed by Miyajima et al., who made a distinction between suprasellar cysts and purely prepontine cystic lesions. The author, based on radiological and anatomic findings, classified these lesions as non-communicating and communicating cysts:

- Intra-arachnoid cyst of the diencephalic Liliequist's membrane (non-communicating cyst);
- Cystic dilation of the interpeduncular cistern (communicating cyst).

As Ozek and Urgun argued, the progressive increase of intra-arachnoid cyst of the diencephalic membrane, can cause a compression of the interpeduncular cistern and dislocate the basilar artery bifurcation behind the posterior wall of the cyst, pushing against the brainstem. Conversely, when cystic dilation of the interpeduncular cistern occurs, the diencephalic membrane would constitute the dome and the mesencephalic membrane the bottom of the cyst. In this latter case, the BA bifurcation would remain inside the cyst. Therefore, since the tip of the basilar artery may be dislocated, its position has to be considered to plan the best approach (Miyajima et al., 2000; Gui et al., 2011; André et aal., 2016; Ozek and Urgun, 2013).

André et al., based on clinical and radiological findings, distinguished 3 main subtypes of SACs, and, according to these subtypes, proposed different therapeutic strategies (Andre et al., 2016) (Figure 1).

SAC-1 includes suprasellar cysts arising from the interpeduncular cistern arachnoid formations, coming from an expansion of the chiasmatic cistern or the diencephalic leaf of the Liliequist membrane, creating mass effect on the third ventricle with early blockage of the foramen of Monro and consequent hydrocephalus.

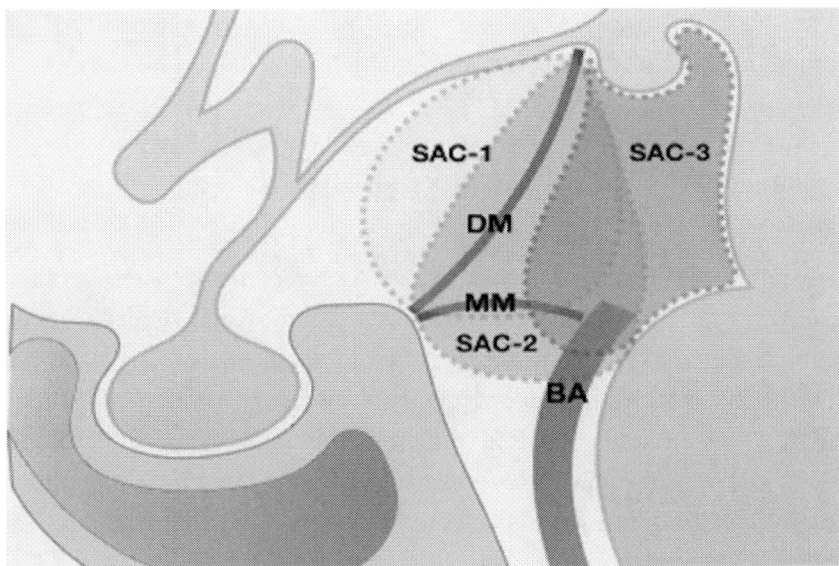

Figure 1. Suprasellar arachnoid cysts classification. SAC-1 is presenting with hydrocephalus. In SAC-2 and SAC-3 the Basilar Artery (BA) is inside the cyst. DM: diencephalic membrane of Liliequist; MM: mesencephalic membrane of Liliequist.

SAC-2 is related to a limited enlargement of the interpeduncular space from a defect of the mesencephalic leaf and the third ventricle remains free, without compression.

SAC-1 and SAC-2 cysts may result in a mass effect on the pituitary stalk creating endocrine disorders. However, the integrity of the diencephalic leaf in SAC-2, may protect from superior expansion. This explain the absence of hydrocephalus in this subtype.

SAC-3 represents asymmetrical forms with involvement of other subarachnoid spaces, mainly lateral sylvian and temporal. They usually present with macrocrania, but only mild or no hydrocephalus. Radiologically, these cysts present an enlargement of the interpeduncular cistern, like SAC-2, but with lateral extension. They may also have a mass effect on the pituitary stalk. However, no endocrinological defects have been reported in this subtype.

In SAC-1 cysts, the basilar tip seems to be moved posteriorly, behind the posterior wall of the cyst.

In SAC-2 and SAC-3, because of the enlargement of the interpeduncular cistern, the basilar bifurcation is included into the cyst.

CLINICAL FEATURES

While initial reports referred mostly to symptomatic patients, mainly presented with hydrocephalus, postmortem studies and modern imaging techniques have highlighted the existence of a majority of incidental ACs. Spontaneous intracystic hemorrhage is a rare complication, which may present with symptoms of raised intracranial pressure or focal neurological deficits and is supposed to be related to a minor trauma with rupture of intracystic or bridging vessels (Iaconetta et al., 2016; Mattox et al., 2010; Kim et al., 2002; Eskandary et al., 2005).

Small SACs are usually silent, requiring only clinical and radiological follow up. Conversely, large ones can exercise mass effect on the adjacent structures, thus causing neurological symptoms (Mustansir et al., 2018). Obstructive hydrocephalus is the most common among the initial signs of suprasellar cysts and develops in almost 90% of patients, especially those who are symptomatic from infancy (Gedikbasi et al., 2010). It may be secondary to an intraventricular, at the foramina of Monro or aqueduct, or extraventricular block, at the level of the tentorial incisura. Obstruction of the intraventricular foramina is usually partial and bilateral, but can occasionally be complete or positional. Hydrocephalus-related symptoms in infants and young children are mostly macrocrania, split sutures, irritability, and developmental delay, whereas in adults they are mainly headache, vomiting, 6th cranial nerve paresis, dizziness, papilloedema, and blurred vision (Juan et al., 2011; Cormac et al., 2011). Approsimately 66% of symptomatic cases occurs with headaches (Helland et al. 2007; Mustansir et al., 2018). Optic nerve involvement, endocrine disfunction, and/or, rarely, a "bobble-head doll" syndrome might be more present in older children and adults (Ozek and Urgun, 2013). Benton et al. described two patients with SAC with the so-called "bobble-head doll" syndrome. They showed repeated head and trunk bowing and head bobbing. However, this syndrome is reported in only 10-16% of patients (Benton et al., 1966; Starzyk et al., 2003). Endocrine disorders include most frequently precocious puberty (IPP) (10-40% of these children, regardless of sex) and less frequently hypothyroidism, hypogonadism, diabetes insipidus, adrenal insufficiency, hyperprolactinemia, and panhypopituitarism. IPP may develop at any prepubertal age, also from the neonatal period but does not seem to be related with the degree of hydrocephalus (Brauner et al., 1987; Pierre-Khan et al., 1990; Hoffman et al., 1982; Woodruff et al., 1987; Starzyk et al., 2003). As reported by Adan et al, endocrinological disorders never regress postoperatively, even when the decrease in the cyst volume is satisfactory and patients require hormone replacement therapies (Adan et al., 2000; Mohn et al., 1999). Erşahin et al. reported that endoscopic treatment of suprasellar arachnoid cysts failed to improve bilateral sixth nerve palsy (Erşahin et al., 2008; Gui et al, 2011). Behavioural disturbances have also been reported to persist postoperatively (Khan and Ahmed, 2017).

DIAGNOSIS

It is now widely accepted that prenatal malformations need careful US and MRI screening during pregnancy. Indeed, less complications have been described for antenatal diagnosed cysts compared to postnatally ones mostly because early diagnosis leads to a precocious treatment (Pierre-Khan et al., 2000).

Only a few cases of prenatal diagnosis of suprasellar cysts have been reported in literature (Gedikbasi et al., 2010; Golash et al., 2001; Diakoumakis et al., 1986; Quinn et al., 1998, Talamonti et al., 2011). Prenatal sonography can show the cyst as a hypoechoic lesion as early as at 20 weeks' gestation. The differential diagnosis for other hypoechoic lesions in the suprasellar region includes epidermoids, Rathke cleft cysts, empty sella, colloid cysts of the third ventricle, ependymal cysts, and cystic neoplasms, such as glioependymal cysts, craniopharyngiomas, cystic pituitary adenomas, and benign cystic gliomas. Suprasellar arachnoid cysts require serial sonographic examination to verify eventual changes in size and exclude obstructive hydrocephalus in utero (Bretelle et al., 2002; Gedikbasi et al, 2010; Pilu et al., 1997). Computerized tomography (CT) scan can also be used to identify haemorrhages, calcifications (not usually present in SACs), or proteinaceous fluid not visible on MRI (Gui et al., 2011; Banna, 1976). André et al. suggested that MRI imaging can easily differentiate the above mentioned subtypes in the prenatal period (André et al., 2016). Before the advent of MRI, most of these cysts were preoperatively evaluated with pneumoencephalography or metrizamide CT ventriculography. These studies also provided valuable information about the CSF dynamics (Gentry et al., 1986). Prenatal MRI helps confirm the diagnosis and exclude other possible central nervous system anomalies, such as, for instance, corpus callosum agenesis and cortical gyral abnormalities. T2-weighted and sagittal CISS images are important to better understand the anatomy and arachnoid adhesions, allowing a more careful preoperative plan, to help in analysing and defining the membranous borders of suprasellar cysts and the position of the basilar artery (Ozek and Urgun, 2013). SACs are visible as non-calcified, well-defined, and non-enhancing lesions with CSF-like signal intensity. Haemorrhagic cysts show varied signal intensity depending on the stage of bleeding and a fluid-blood level can be visualized into the cyst. As mentioned, SACs can cause the occlusion of foramen or foramina of Monro giving the typical "Mickey Mouse appearance" on axial MRI for dilated third and lateral ventricles. MRI also helps the differential diagnosis. For instance, epidermoids show the characteristic diffusion restriction and the typical enhancement of their solid component. Moreover, gadolinium-enhanced MRI allows also the differentiation with cystic neoplasms, infections (tuberculosis, neurocysticercosis), or inflammatory cysts (granulomatous process) (Mattox et al., 2010; Wiener et al., 1987). Wang et al described few radiological signs of SACs on MRI: the upward displacement of the optic chiasm and the ventral brainstem displacement. Suprasellar cysts could be misdiagnosed as a dilated third ventricle due to aqueductal stenosis and MRI can help to differentiate showing the typical upward deviation of the mammillary bodies, instead of a downward displacement, as for dilated third ventricle. As well, a posterior brainstem displacement is present when there is a retroclival development of the cyst (Crimmins et al., 2006; Wang et al., 2004). Cine-phase contrast MRI is useful to study CSF flow dynamics. By convention, anterior flow is hypointense and posterior flow is hyperintense. The most crucial diagnostic information to look for are: whether the cyst communicates with the subarachnoid space; the presence, severity, and location of intraventricular CSF obstruction; and the presence of eventual extraventricular CSF block (Yildiz et al., 2005; Santamarta et al., 1995).

Although modern imaging modalities are considered important complementary tools investigation for reaching a differential diagnosis, the histological examination remains mandatory (Miyagami et al., 1993).

Furthermore, fetal arachnoid cysts can be associated with chromosomal abnormalities. Therefore, prenatal diagnosis, especially when associated with other abnormalities, should undergo cytogenetic investigations (Caemaert et al., 1992).

TREATMENT

Surgical indications should consider the presence of signs or symptoms such as increased ICP, visual disturbances, and/or evolving cysts. Endocrine and behavioural dysfunctions are not an indication for surgery because, as previously mentioned, they never regress postoperatively (Adan et al., 2000; Crimmins et al., 2006). In order to consider a possible surgical option, it is necessary to understand if SACs are responsible or not for the presenting disorders, especially in case of common symptoms such as headache (Al-Holou et al., 2010). Therefore, Choi et al. divided these cystic lesions in three categories, based on clinical presentation and reasons for surgery. The first group included SACs presenting with hydrocephalus and intracranial hypertension. In the second group, cysts aroused with vague symptoms such as headache, large head, skull abnormalities, strabismus, seizures, and developmental delays. A third group was characterized by minimal or no clinical symptoms. The authors reported an improvement rate only in the first group; conversely, a minimal and partial improvement was seen in the second and third group, respectively (Choi et al., 2015). Spontaneous resolution of SACs at routine MRIs has been documented, which reinforces the concept that asymptomatic patients should not be operated (Choi et al., 2015; Dodd et al., 2002).

Based on André et al. classification, the recognition of the different subtypes might be helpful for the choice of the best treatment option.

SACs-1 become rapidly symptomatic due to hydrocephalus and intracranial hypertension, therefore requiring surgical treatment as soon as possible. Endoscopy is nowadays the treatment of choice in these cysts with an expected favourable outcome.

SACs-2 are mostly diagnosed antenatally or incidentally and might remain stable and asymptomatic, without requiring a surgical treatment. However, a minority of these cysts increase in size, having a mass effect and therefore requiring a surgical treatment.

SACs-3 are characterized by mild hydrocephalus associated to macrocrania. Indeed, these cysts tend to enlarge over time, thus requiring a treatment when they become symptomatic. The ipsilateral pterional approach has been proposed as the primary treatment for asymmetrical SAC-3, but endoscopy may play a role too (Talamonti et al., 2011).

Instead, a minimally invasive open marsupialization has been described as an adequate alternative to endoscopy for both symptomatic SAC-2 and SAC-3 (Gui et al., 2011).

Before the advent of endoscopy, open surgery was considered the gold standard for SACs management (Boutarbouch et al., 2008). Nowadays, in the presence of tiny ventricles, it has still a crucial role. Various open surgical procedures have been described for suprasellar cysts, including subfrontal, subtemporal, transcallosal, and transsphenoidal approaches (Cormac et al., 2011; Shim et al., 2009; Murali et al., 1979; Rappaport et al., 1993).

Potential complications for open procedures include meningitis, neurological deficits, cranial nerves injuries, CSF leakage, seizures, subdural collections, and even the need for more than one surgical treatment after the failure of an initial decompression. Limitations of the endonasal approach, such as dural closure difficulties, risk of infection, and CSF leaks, especially in intradural surgeries, are well known (Shim et al., 2009).

Cystoperitoneal, ventriculoperitoneal, or cystoventricular shunts are the most common options when shunting is placed. Placement of lumboperitoneal shunting was reported but its use is controversial because of the risk of central herniation (Germano et al., 2003; Berlis et al., 2006; Behrens et al., 1993). Boutarbouch et al. described a cystosubdural shunting as an efficient and safe minimally invasive technique for the treatment of supratentorial arachnoid cysts (Boutarbouch et al., 2008). Moreover, a Rickham reservoir attached to a ventricular catheter which drain both the cyst and the ventricles have been used when there is no communicating hydrocephalus, but a high failure rate was reported (Mattox et al., 2010). Common problems with any shunting procedure, such as shunt malfunction, infection, overdrainage, and shunt dependency are widely described (Juan et al., 2011; Cormac et al., 2011; Al-Holou et al., 2010; Christian et al, 2006; Martinez-Lage et al., 2009). Shim et al. tried to identify factors related to the shunt-dependency and found correlations with younger age at shunting, lower pressure of the valve, longer follow-up duration, and larger initial size of the cyst (Shim et al., 2009).

Moreover, the success rate of shunting as a definitive treatment for SACs is reported to be only 10% (Yadav et al., 2010). In fact, the cyst might remain distended and continue to exert mass effect over thalamic, hypotalamo-hypophyseal, and optic structures (Brauner et al., 1987).

Guzel et al. proposed the use of a stereotactic cystoventriculostomy by catheter implantation. This procedure has been proposed as an alternative option to open cyst fenestration and cystoperitoneal shunting, leading to complete resolution of clinical symptoms. However, because of the cyst's wall toughness, the catheter can deviate without penetrating the cyst (Guzel et al., 2007; Behrens et al., 1993; D'Angelo et al., 1999).

Endoscopic surgery of SACs enables the surgeon to achieve decompression of the cyst with direct visualization and minimizing the risks of injuries (Cappabianca et al., 2002; Cavallo et al., 2008; Cinalli et al., 2005). It is an extremely well-tolerated procedure, even in very young children, allowing a shunt-free existence (El-Ghandour et al., 2011). Surgical morbidity seems to be very low and acceptable compared with other types of treatment modalities (Di Rocco et al., 2005; Gangemi et al., 2011). It has an additional advantage of identification and treatment of ventricular abnormality, such as foramen of Monro stenosis and cerebral aqueduct occlusion. Therefore, an endoscopic fenestration of the wall from the lateral ventricle has been advocated as best strategy and represents the actual primary treatment for SACs (Gangemi et al., 2011). A success rate of up to 71–90% has been documented (Gangemi et al., 2011, Gui et al., 2011). Furthermore, endoscopic treatment dramatically reduces operative time other that surgical morbidity compared with craniotomy (Yadav et al., 2010). In the presence of tiny ventricles, endoscopy might be impractical and open marsupialization of the cyst into the basal cisterns has been suggested over shunt insertion to avoid the risk of shunt dependency (Crimmins et al., 2006). Shunting can be a useful secondary treatment in recurrent cases.

The main actual debate around the endoscopic treatment includes the type of surgery and the results of a second endoscopic procedures following the failure of a previous one (Crimmins et al., 2006). The ventriculocistostomy (VC technique) involves fenestration of the apical membrane, usually at the level of the foramen of Monro, between the ventricle and the cyst (Gui et al., 2011). The ventriculocystocisternostomy (VCC technique) involves fenestration of both the apical membrane into the ventricle and the basal membrane into the prepontine cistern (Cormac et al., 2011). Crimmins et al. reported a higher success rate in patients treated with VCC (100%) then those managed with VC technique (25%) (Crimmins et al., 2006). A similar outcome between VCC and VC techniques was described by McCrea et al., Kim et al., and by Maher et al. who associated VC with a higher rate of reintervention, 20% vs 9% in VCC. Gangemi et al. revealed a higher rate of clinical and radiological improvement after VCC (94,3%) than after VC (85,7%) (McCrea et al., 2015; Kim et al., 1999; Kim et al., 2017; Maher et al., 2011; Gangemi et al., 2007). Gui et al. tried to explain the origin of these results and concluded that VC might be used for communicating cysts, while VCC should be suitable for non-communicating ones (Gui et al., 2011). Rangel-Castilla et al. reported aqueductal obstruction as a possible cause of VC failure. Therefore, in the case of aqueductal occlusion, VCC would be the best treatment (Rangel-Castilla et al., 2009). Paris group reported that the success rate of primary endoscopic surgery, although not statistically significant, was higher for VCC (85%) than for VC (57%) (Crimmins et al., 2006). Buxton described the use of a flexible endoscope and found it particularly advantageous because, when decompressing the cyst, the anatomy moves. He considered VCC unnecessary because the opening of the cyst roof into the ventricular system would be sufficient to restore the flow through the aqueduct (Buxton et al., 1999). However, it has been reported that the superior fenestration tends to close, regardless of whether a single or dual fenestration is performed, because stretching of the third ventricle creates excess tissue that can overlap and seal the fenestration after the operation. The persistence of the basal opening, when facing a secondary closure of the apical fenestration, allows adequate cyst decompression into the basal cisterns, thus decreasing the risk of recurrence (Decq et al., 1996). Moreover, Sood et al. reported that VCC associated to the radical shrinkage of the cyst by using bipolars might prevent the aqueduct obstruction and the closure of the cyst opening (Sood et al., 2005).

Many microsurgical techniques have been described, from complete the resection of the cyst's wall to the simple marsupialization (Jones et al., 1989; Konovalov et al., 1988; Raimondi et al., 1980). However, because of the anatomical relationships between the membrane and the underlying neural tissues, authors recommended a selective opening of the basal cisterns with an incomplete resection of the outer cyst wall (André et al., 2016). An extensive resection of the dome of the SAC when invaginated into the third ventricle and firmly adherent to the hypothalamus can cause transient or persistent diabetes insipidus after surgery (Gentry, 1986). Fenestrations have shown better results when dual and larger (approximately 10-15 mm). To verify that the floor has been perforated, identification of the abducens nerve is crucial after the procedure, the cyst should become a "tent-like structure", and the compression on surrounding structures should resolve (Yadav et al., 2010; Mustansir et al., 2018; Ogiwara et al., 2011).

Opening of the cyst has been described by using bipolar, monopolar, laser (Pierre-Khan et al., 1990; Caemert et al., 1992), or by using a balloon-mounted stent through an endoscopic approach (Berlis et al., 2006).

Once intracranial pressure is normalized and normal CSF flow dynamics are restored, ex vacuo ventriculomegaly may persist and does not necessarily require treatment in the absence of symptoms (Mattox et al., 2010). However, cases with progressive hydrocephalus despite cyst reduction are possible (Talamonti et al., 2011).

CASE SERIES

A series of 18 suprasellar arachnoid cysts were consecutively enrolled at Niguarda Hospital, Milan, by a dedicated team over a 15-year period.

History was obtained including sex, age at presentation, eventual previous trauma or surgery, clinical signs and symptoms, endocrinological and ophtalmological investigations were recorded, and treatment strategy and postoperative complications and follow-up were listed. Ventricular and cyst size were monitored during the follow-up.

Indications for surgery included symptoms of raised ICP, visual deterioration, or enlargement of the cyst for asymptomatic patients. A conservative treatment was proposed for asymptomatic patients with stable cysts and with an isolated endocrinal dysfunction.

All patients underwent preoperative MRI. Six of them underwent CT scan at arrival followed by MRI and 11 patients performed MRI as a first exam. One patient was diagnosed in the prenatal period at the ultrasonography second trimester study. Then, he was followed with routine foetal US and MRI and repeated MRI at birth. In this case the progressive enlargement of SAC-3 was documented by repeated foetal

MRI and the patient had been operated in the early neonatal period by an endoscopic approach. Postoperatively, as aforementioned, the cyst decreased but hydrocephalus developed (Talamonti et al., 2011).

We used the André et al. classification in three subtypes: 12 patients had SAC-1, 4 patients had SAC-2, and 2 patients had SAC-3 (André et al., 2016). Hydrocephalus was noted at presentation in all the SAC-1 patients, and developed postoperatively in one SAC-3 patient.

Of the 18 patients treated, 10 were male and 8 females, with ages ranging from 1 month to 31 years (mean 6.8 years). No trauma at delivery were reported. The most frequent presenting symptom was headache in nine patients, in three patient macrocrania, in one patient head bobbing, and in one patient developmental delay. In four cases, indication for surgery consisted of progressive cyst increase (3 children and 1 adult). Associated endocrinological dysfunctions were not found in any cases.

At the preoperative MRI, optic chiasm deviation, displacement of the mammillary bodies, and brainstem compression were present in all patients.

Endoscopic surgery with ventriculocystocisternostomy was the primary treatment in all cases, using rigid endoscope, bipolar coagulation and, more recently, a laser beam, and balloon catheter for the enlargement of the stoma. Neuronavigation was helpful when the anatomy was very distorted.

The floor of the third ventricle was widely opened into the roof of the cyst, and then the inferior wall was widely fenestrated into the prepontine cistern observing the pulsation of the free edges of the cyst. Intraoperatively, a valve-like mechanism was observed in all SAC-2 cases where the basilar artery was entering the cyst through the inferior wall.

No endoscopic treatment had to be converted to open surgery; no mortality or permanent morbidity were reported. One patient (5.5%) with a SAC-3 cyst required a second procedure with a ventriculoperitoneal shunt because of progressive hydrocephalus.

Follow-up ranged from 1 to 15 years, with a mean of 80 months. Of all patients, 94.5% achieved a clinical improvement, one (5.5%) remained clinically stable during follow-up not improving his IQ after surgery. Each patient had a postoperative cine-phase MRI showing an improved CSF dynamic. Cyst decreases or even disappearances were documented in all cases and there was no cyst recurrence (Figures 2-4).

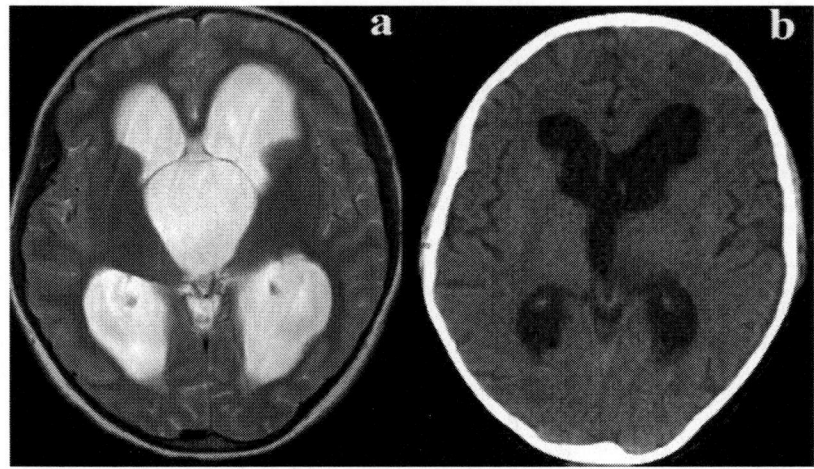

Figure 2. Preoperative Axial MRI (a) and Postoperative Axial CT scan (b) of SAC-1.

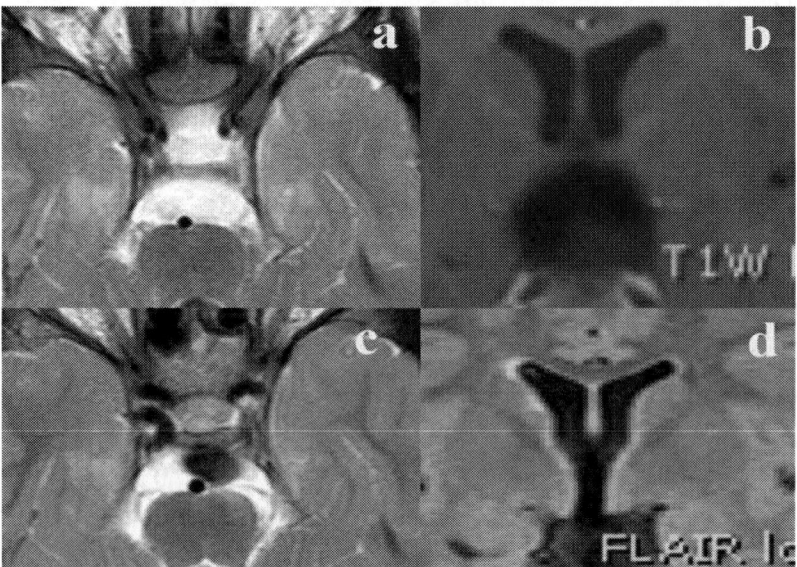

Figure 3. Preoperative Axial (a) and Coronal (b), Postoperative Axial (c) and Coronal (d) MR images of SAC-2.

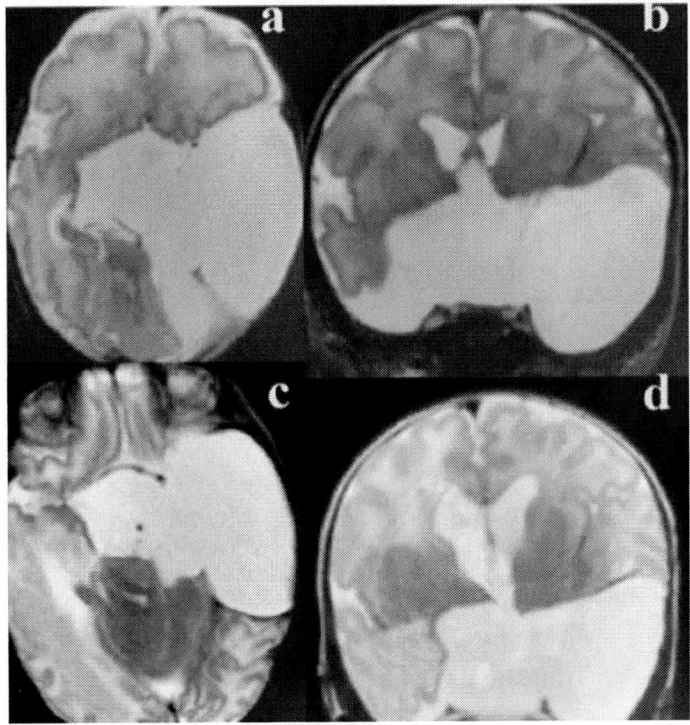

Figure 4. Preoperative Axial (a) and Coronal (b), Postoperative Axial (c) and Coronal (d) MR images of SAC-3.

Accordingly, the endoscopic dual cyst fenestration was then successful in 17 (95.5%) of 18 cases.

CONCLUSION

Surgery is recommended in patients with increasing ICP, visual disturbances, and/or evolving cysts. Endocrine disturbances alone are not an indication for surgery because they always persist after surgery. Endoscopic dual fenestration is the best treatment, with a good overall clinical and radiological outcome, and can be considered as a minimally invasive, safe, and effective procedure.

REFERENCES

Adan L, Bussières L, Dinand V, Zerah M, Pierre-Kahn A, Brauner R. (2000). "Growth, puberty and hypothalamic-pituitary function in children with suprasellar arachnoid cyst." *Eur J Pediatr,* 159:348–55.

Adeeb N, Deep A, Griessenauer J, Mortazavi M, Watanabe K, Loukas M, Tubbs R, Cohen-Gadol A. (2013). "The intracranial arachnoid matter." *Childs Nerv Syst,* 29:17-33.

Al-Holou WN, Yew AY, Boomsaad ZE, Garton HJ, Muraszko KM, Maher CO. (2010). "Prevalence and natural history of arachnoid cysts in children." *J Neurosurg Pediatr,* 5:578-85.

Albuquerque FC, Giannotta SL. (1997). "Arachnoid cyst rupture producing subdural hygroma and intracranial hypertension: case reports." *Neurosurgery,* 41:951-55.

André A, Zerah M, Roujeau T, Brunelle F, Blauwblomme T, Puget S, Bourgeois M, Sainte-Rose C, Ville Y, Di Rocco F. (2016). "Suprasellar Arachnoid Cysts: toward a new simple classification based on prognosis and treatment modality." *Neurosurgery,* 78:370-80.

Banna M. (1976). "Arachnoid cysts on computed tomography." *Am J Roentgenol,* 127:979–82.

Barlow A. (1935). "Suprasellar arachnoid cyst." *Arch Ophthalmol,* 14:53-60.

Behrens P, Ostertag CB. (1993). "Stereotactic management of congenital midline cysts." *Acta Neurochir,* 123:141-46.

Benton JW, Nellhaus G, Huttenlocher PR. (1996). "The bobble-head doll syndrome. Report of a unique truncal tremor associated with third ventricular cyst and hydrocephalus in children." *Neurology,* 16:725-29.

Berlis A, Vesper J, Ostertag C. "Stent placement for intracranial cysts by combined stereotactic/endoscopic surgery." (2006). *Neurosurgery,* 59:474–80.

Binitie O, Williams B, Case CP. (1984). "A suprasellar subarachnoid pouch; aetiological considerations." *J Neurol Neurosurg Psychiatry,* 47:1066-74.

Boutarbouch M, El Ouahabi A, Rifi L, Arkha Y, Derraz S, El Khamlichi A. (2008). "Management of intracranial arachnoid cysts: Institutional experience with initial 32 cases and review of the literature." *Clinical Neurology and neurosurgery,* 110:1-7.

Bretelle F, Senat MV, Bernard JP, Hillion Y, Ville Y. (2002). "First trimester diagnosis of fetal arachnoid cyst: prenatal implication." *Ultrasound Obstet Gynecol,* 20:400–02.

Brauner R, Pierre-Kahn A, Nemedy-Sandor E, Rappaport R, Hirsch JF. (1987). "Pubertes precoces par kyste arachnoidien suprasellaire. Analyse de 6 observations." *Arch Fr Pediatr,* 44:489-93.

Bright R. (1831). "Serous cysts in the arachnoid. Report of medical cases selected with a view of illustrating the symptoms and cure of diseases by a reference to morbid anatomy." *Diseases of the brain and nervous system.*

Caemaert J, Abdullah J, Calliauw L, Carton D, Dhooge C, van Coster R. (1992). "Endoscopic treatment of suprasellar arachnoid cysts." *Acta Neurochir (Wien),* 119:68–73.

Buxton N, Vloeberghs M, Punt J. (1999). "Technical note. Flexible neuroendoscope treatment of suprasellar arachnoid cysts." *British Journal of Neurosurgery,* 13: 316-18.

Cappabianca P, Cavallo LM, Colao A, Del Basso De Caro M, Esposito F, Cirillo S, Lombardi G, de Divitiis E. (2002). "Endoscopic endonasal transsphenoidal approach: outcome analysis of 100 consecutive procedures." *Minim Invasive Neurosurg,* 45:193–200.

Cavallo LM, Prevedello D, Esposito F, Laws ER Jr, Dusick JR, Messina A, Jane JA, Kelly DF, Cappabianca P. (2008). "The role of the endoscope in the transsphenoidal management of cystic lesions of the sellar region." *Neurosurg Rev,* 31:55–64.

Choi JW, Lee JY, Phi JH, Kim SK, Wang KC. (2015). "Stricter indications are recommended for fenestration surgery in intracranial arachnoid cysts of children." *Child Nerv Syst,* 31:77-86.

Christian AH, Wester K. (2006). "Arachnoid cysts in adults: longterm follow-up of patients treated with internal shunts to the subdural compartment." *Surg Neurol,* 66:56–61.

Cinalli G, Cappabianca P, de Falco R, Spennato P, Cianciulli E, Cavallo LM, Esposito F, Ruggiero C, Maggi G, de Divitiis E. (2005). "Current state and future development of intracranial neuroendoscopic surgery." *Expert Rev Med Devices,* 2:351-73.

Cormac O, Maher and Goumnerova L. (2011). "The effectiveness of ventriculocystocisternostomy for suprasellar arachnoid cysts." *J Neurosurg Pediatrics,* 7:64-72.

Crimmins DW, Pierre-Kahn A, Sainte-Rose C, Zerah M. (2006). "Treatment of suprasellar cysts and patient outcome." *J Neurosurg,* 105:107–14.

D'Angelo V, Gorgoglione L, Catapano G. (1999). "Treatment of symptomatic intracranial arachnoid cysts by stereotactic cyst-ventricular shunting." *Stereotact Funct Neurosurg,* 72:62–9.

Decq P, Brugieres P, Le Guerinel C, Djindjian M, Keravel Y, Nguyen JP. (1996). "Percutaneous endoscopic treatment of suprasellar arachnoid cysts: ventriculocystostomy or ventriculocystocisternostomy? Technical note." *J Neurosurg,* 84:696–701.

Di Rocco F, Yoshino M, Oi S. (2005). "Neuroendoscopic transventricular ventriculocystostomy in treatment for intracranial cysts." *J Neurosurg,* 103:54-60.

Diakoumakis EE, Weinberg B, Mollin J. (1986). "Prenatal sonographic diagnosis of a suprasellar arachnoid cyst." *J Ultrasound Med,* 5:529-30.

Dodd RL, Barnes PD, Huhn SL. (2002). "Spontaneous resolution of a prepontine arachnoid cyst. Case report and review of the literature." *Pediatr Neurosurg,* 37:152-7.

Du Boulay GH. (1966). "Pulsatile movements in the CSF pathways." *Br.J. Radiol,* 39:255-62.

Du Boulay GH, J. O'Connell, J. Currie, T. Bostick, P. Verity. (1972). "Further Investigations on pulsatile movements in the cerebros pinal fluid pathways." *Acta Radiol,* 13:496–523.

El-Ghandour NM. (2011). "Endoscopic treatment of suprasellar arachnoid cysts in children." *J Neurosurg Pediatr,* 8:6-14.

Erşahin Y, Kesikçi H, Rüksen M, Aydin C, Mutluer S. (2008). "Endoscopic treatment of suprasellar arachnoid cysts." *Childs Nerv Syst,* 24:1013-20.

Eskandary H, Sabba M, Khajehpour F, Eskandari M. (2005). "Incidental findings in brain computed tomography scans of 3000 head trauma patients." *Surg Neurol,* 63:550–53.

Fox JL, Al-Mefty O. (1980). "Suprasellar arachnoid cysts: an extension of the membrane of Liliequist." *Neurosurg,* 7:615-618.

Froelich SC, Abdel Aziz KM, Cohen PD, van Loveren HR, Keller JT. (2008). "Microsurgical and endoscopic anatomy of Liliequist's membrane: a complex and variable structure of the basal cisterns." *Neurosurgery,* 63:1-9.

Gangemi M, Colella G, Magro F, Maiuri F. (2007). "Suprasellar arachnoid cysts: endoscopy versus microsurgical cyst excision and shunting." *Br J Neurosurg,* 21:276-80.

Gedikbasi A., Palabiyik F, Oztarhan A, Yildirim G, Eren C, Ozyurt SS, Ceylan Y. (2010). "Prenatal diagnosis of a suprasellar arachnoid cyst with 2- and 3-dimensional sonography and fetal magnetic resonance imaging." *J Ultrasound Med,* 29:1487-93.

Gentry LR, Menezes AH, Turski PA, Smoker WR, Cornell SH, Ramirez L. (1986). "Suprasellar arachnoid cysts 2. Evaluation of CSF dynamics." *Am J Neuroradiol,* 7:87-96.

Germano A, Caruso G, Caffo M, Baldari S, Calisto A, Meli F. (2003). "The treatment of large supratentorial arachnoid cysts in infants with cyst-peritoneal shunting and Hakim programmable valve." *Childs Nerv Syst,* 19:166–73.

Go KG, Houthoff HJ, Blaauw EH, Havinga P, Hartsuiker J. (1984). "Arachnoid cysts of the sylvian fissure. Evidence of fluid secretion." *J Neurosurg,* 60:803-13.

Golash A, Mitchell G, Mallucci C, May P, Pilling D. (2001). "Prenatal diagnosis of suprasellar arachnoid cyst and postnatal endoscopic treatment." *Childs Nerv Syst,* 17:739-42.

Gui SB, Wang XS, Zhang XZ, Li CZ. (2011). "Suprasellar cysts: Clinical presentation, surgical indications, and optimal surgical treatment." *BMC Neurology*, 11:52.

Guzel A, Ostertage CB, Trippel M. (2007). "Suprasellar arachnoid cyst: a 20-year follow-up after stereotactic internal drainage: Case report and review of the literature." *Turkish Neurosurgery*, 3:211-18.

Helland CA, Lund-Johansen M, Wester K. (2010). "Location, sidedness, and sex distribution of intracranial arachnoid cysts in a population based sample." *J Neurosurg*, 113:934–39.

Hoffman HJ, Hendrick EB, Humphreys RP, Armstrong EA. (1982). "Investigation and management of suprasellar arachnoid cysts." *J Neurosurg*, 57:597–602.

Iaconetta G, Esposito M, Maiuri F, Cappabianca P. (2006). "Arachnoid cyst with intracystic haemorrhage and subdural haematoma: case report and literature review." *Neurol Sci*, 6:451-55.

Invergo.D, Tomita T. (2012). "De novo suprasellar arachnoid cyst: case report and review of the literature." *Pediatr Neurosurg*, 48:199-203.

Jones RF, Warnock TH, Nayanar V, Gupta JM. (1989). "Suprasellar arachnoid cysts: management by cyst wall resection." *Neurosurgery*, 25:554–61.

Martinez-Lage JF, Pérez-Espejo MA, Almagro MJ, Lopez Guerrero AL. (2011). "Hydrocephalus and arachnoid cysts" *Childs Nerv Syst*, 27:1643-52.

Kasdon DL, Douglas EA, Broughan MF. (1977). "Suprasellar arachnoid cyst diagnosed preoperatively by computerized tomographic scanning." *Surg Neurol*, 7:299-303.

Khan AH, Ahmed SE. (2017). "Arachnoid cyst and psychosis." *Cureus*, 21:e1707.

Kim BS, Illes J, Kaplan RT, Reiss A, Atlas SW. (2002). "Incidental findings on pediatric MR images of the brain." *AJNR*, 23:1674–77.

Kim MH. (1999). "The role of endoscopic fenestration procedures for cerebral arachnoid cysts." *J Korean Med Sci*, 14:443–47.

Kim MH. (2017). "Transcortical endoscopic surgery for intraventricular lesions." *J Korean Neurosurg*, 60:327-34.

Konovalov AN, Rostotskaia VI, Ivakina NI, Simernitskii BP. (1988). "Surgical treatment of suprasellar cerebrospinal fluid cysts." *Zh Vopr Neirokhir*, 1:11-16.

Krawchenko J, Collins GH. (1979). "Pathology of an arachnoid cyst." *J Neurosurg*, 50:224-28.

Lewis AJ. (1962). "Infantile hydrocephalus caused by arachnoid cyst. Case report." *J Neurosurg*, 19:431-4.

Maher CO, Goumnerova L. (2011). "The effectiveness of ventriculocystocisternostomy for suprasellar arachnoid cysts." *J Neurosurg Pediatr*, 7:64-72.

Martínez-Lage JF, Ruíz-Espejo AM, Almagro MJ, Alfaro R, Felipe-Murcia M, López-Guerrero AL. (2009). "CSF overdrainage in shunted intracranial arachnoid cysts: a series and review." *Childs Nerv Syst*, 25:1061–69.

Mattox A, Choi JD, Leith-Gray L, Grant GA, Adamson DC. (2010). "Guidelines for the management of obstructive hydrocephalus from suprasellar-prepontine arachnoid cysts using endoscopic third ventriculocystocisternostomy." *Surgical Innovation*, 17:206-16.

McCrea HJ, George E, Settler A, Schwartz TH, Greenfield JP. (2015). "Pediatric suprasellar tumors." *Journal of Child Neurology*, 1-10.

Miyagami M, Tsubokawa T. (1993). "Histological and ultrastructural finding of benign intracranial cysts." *Noshuyo Byori*, 10:151–60.

Miyajima M, Arai H, Okuda O, Hishii M, Nakanishi H, Sato K. (2000) "Possible origin of suprasellar arachnoid cysts: neuroimaging and neurosurgical observations in nine cases." *J Neurosurg*, 93:62-7.

Mohn A, Schoof E, Fahlbusch R, Wenzel D, Dörr HG. (1999). "The endocrine spectrum of arachnoid cysts in childhood." *Pediatr Neurosurg*, 31:316–21.

Murali R, Epstein F. (1979). "Diagnosis and treatment of suprasellar arachnoid cyst. Report of three cases." *J Neurosurg*, 50:515–18.

Mustansir F, Bashir S, Darbar A. "Management of Arachnoid Cysts. A comprehensive Review." *Cureus* 10(4):e2458

Ogiwara H, Morota N, Joko M, Hirota K. (2011). "Endoscopic fenestrations for suprasellar arachnoid cysts." *J Neurosurg Pediatr,* 8:484-88.

Ozek MM, Urgun K. (2013). "Neuroendoscopic management of suprasellar arachnoid cysts." *World Neurosurg,* 79:S19e3-e8.

Pierre-Kahn A, Capelle L, Braunner R. (1990). "Presentation and management of suprasellar arachnoid cysts. Review of 20 cases." *J Neurosurg,* 73:355–59.

Pierre-Kahn A, Hanlo P, Sonigo P, Parisot D, McConnell RS. (2000). "The contribution of prenatal diagnosis to the understanding of malformative intracranial cysts: state of the art." *Childs Nerv Syst,* 16:619-26.

Pilu G, Falco P, Perolo A, Sandri F, Cocchi G, Ancora G, Bovicelli L. (1997). "Differential diagnosis and outcome of intracranial hypoechoic lesions: report of 21 cases." *Ultrasound Obstet Gynecol,* 9:229–236.

Quinn TM, Hubbard AM, Adzick NS. (1998). "Prenatal magnetic resonance imaging enhances fetal diagnosis." *J Pediatr Surg,* 33:553–58.

Raimondi AJ, Shimoji T, Gutierrez FA. (1980). "Suprasellar cysts: surgical treatment and results." *Childs Brain,* 7:57-72.

Rangel-Castilla L, Torres-Corzo J, Vecchia RR, Mohanty A, Nauta HJ. (2009). "Coexistent intraventricular abnormalities in periventricular giant arachnoid cysts." *J Neurosurg Pediatr,* 3:225-31.

Rappaport ZH. (1993). "Suprasellar arachnoid cysts: options in operative management." *Acta Neurochir,* 122:71–5.

Rengachary SS, Watanabe I. (1981). "Ultrastructure and pathogenesis of intracranial arachnoid cysts." *J Neuropathol Exp Neurol,* 40:61–83.

Sandberg DI, McComb JG, Krieger MD. (2005). "Chemical analysis of fluid obtained from intracranial arachnoid cysts in pediatric patients." *J Neurosurg,* 103:427-32.

Santamarta D, Aguas J, Ferree E. (1995). "The natural history of Arachnoid Cysts: Endoscopic and Cine-Mode MRI Evidence of a Slit-Valve Mechanism." *Minim Invas Neurosurg,* 38:133-37.

Schachenmayr W, Friede RL. (1979). "Fine structure of arachnoid cysts." *J Neuropathol Exp Neurol*, 38:434–46.

Schroeder HWS, Gaab MR. (1997). "Endoscopic observation of a slit-valve mechanism in a suprasellar prepontine arachnoid cyst: case report." *Neurosurgery,* 40:198–200.

Shim KW, Lee YH, Park EK, Park YS, Choi JU, Kim DS. (2009). "Treatment option for arachnoid cysts." *Childs Nerv Syst,* 25:1459-66.

Sood S, Schulmann MU, Cakan N, Ham SD. (2005). "Endoscopic fenestration and coagulation shrinkage of suprasellar arachnoid cysts. Technical note." *J Neurosurg,* 102:127-33.

Starkman SP, Brown TC, Linell EA. (1958). "Cerebral arachnoid cysts." *J Neuropathol Exp Neurol*, 17:484–500.

Starzyk J, Kwiatkowski S, Wieslav U, Starzyk B, Harasiewicz M, Kalicka-Kasperczyk A, Tylek-Lemanska D, Dziatkowiak H. (2003). "Suprasellar arachnoidal cyst as a cause of precocious puberty- Report of three patients and literature overview. *Journal of Pediatric Endocrinology and Metabolism,* 16:447-55.

Talamonti G, D'Aliberti G, Picano M, Debernardi A, Collice M. (2011). "Intracranial cysts containing cerebrospinal fluid-like fluid: results of endoscopic neurosurgery in a series of 64 consecutive cases." *Neurosurgery,* 68:788–803.

Wang JC, Heier L, Souweidane MM. (2004). "Advances in the endoscopic management of suprasellar arachnoid cysts in children." *J Neurosurg,* 100:418–26.

Wiener SN, Pearlstein AE, Eiber A. (1987). "MR imaging of intracranial arachnoid cysts." *J Comput Assist Tomogr,* 11:236–41.

Williams.B, Guthkelch AN. (1974). "Why do central arachnoid pouches expand?" *J Neurol Neurosurg Psych,* 37:1085-92.

Woodruff WW, Heinz ER, Djang WT, Voorhees D. (1987). "Hyperprolactinemia: an unusual manifestation of suprasellar cystic lesions." *Am J Neuroradiol,* 8:113-16.

Yadav YR, Parihar V, Sinha M, Jain N. (2010). "Endoscopic treatment of the suprasellar arachnoid cyst." *Neurology India,* 58:280-3.

Yildiz H, Erdogan C, Yalcin R, Yazici, Hakyemez B, Parlak M, Tuncel E. (2005). "Evaluation of communication between intracranial arachnoid cysts and cisterns with phase-contrast cine MR imaging." *Am J Neuroradiol, 26*:145-51.

In: Neuroendoscopic Procedures …
Editor: Soner Duru

ISBN: 978-1-68507-092-2
© 2021 Nova Science Publishers, Inc.

Chapter 7

NEUROENDOSCOPIC CHALLENGES IN THE TREATMENT OF VENTRICULAR TUMORS

Piero Andrea Oppido[*], *MD, PhD*

Department of Neurosurgery,
IRCCS Regina Elena National Cancer Institute, Rome, Italy

ABSTRACT

Neuroendoscopy is presently considered a scarcely invasive surgical approach for expanding lesions bulging into the ventricle, as a relevant tool in performing bioptic procedures, discontinuation of cystic walls or tumor removal in selected cases. Furthermore, the diffusion of neuroimaging and the accurate follow-up of brain tumor patients have more frequently allowed to document tumoral and pseudo-tumoral cystic areas causing the obstruction of cerebrospinal fluid (CSF) pathways. Neuroendoscopic procedures enable fenestration of cystic lesions, in addition to third ventriculostomy or septostomy in order to restore CSF pathways.

---

[*] Corresponding Author's E-mail: piero.oppido@ifo.gov.it.

In this study, we evaluate our experience regarding 96 patients affected with brain tumors arising from the wall of the third or lateral ventricle. Hydrocephalus or obstruction of CSF flow was present in all our cases. The endoscopic technique, septostomy, cystostomy, third ventriculostomy (ETV) or tumor resection were alone or simultaneously performed to control intracranial hypertension.

The ETV was carried out in 68 patients with non-communicating hydrocephalus. In 6 LG astrocytoma the ETV was the only definite surgical treatment. In 20 cystic tumors, cystostomy and marsupialization into the ventricle solved a relevant mass effect with clinical intracranial hypertension syndrome. In 12 patients, neuroendoscopic relief of CSF pathways by septostomy associated with Ommaya reservoir or one catheter shunt was possible. Removal was possible in 6 colloid cysts and 5 cystic craniopharyngiomas by restoring CSF flow without other procedures. After intracranial hypertension control, in 28 malignant gliomas, 18 with metastases or leptomeningeal carcinomatosis and 6 with lymphomas were allowed to continue tumor adjuvant therapy ameliorating the quality of life. In 6 cystic central neurocytomas and 12 ependymomas subsequent microsurgical removal was achieved. Other tumors included PNET, pinealoblastoma, radionecrosis and epidermoid cyst, malignant teratoma.

Neuroendoscopy was found to be safe and effective, avoiding major surgical approaches and without any relevant post-operative morbidity, due to its mininvasive characteristics and reduced complications. Based on these results and on the increasing series described in the literature, endoscopic techniques should be considered the selected approach in treating CSF obstructions by para-intraventricular tumors. This surgical procedure is not limited to relief of non-communicating hydrocephalus, but it is also useful for tumor removal or biopsies and evacuation of cystic lesions. In patients affected by malignant tumors, neuroendoscopy can be performed to control intracranial hypertension before starting adjuvant chemotherapy or radiotherapy.

Keywords: ventricular tumor, endoscopic biopsy, endoscopic third ventriculostomy, hydrocephalus

INTRODUCTION

Intraventricular and paraventricular tumors are rare lesions occluding often the normal (CSF) pathways. They present a diagnostic challenge for the surgeon because of a broad differential diagnosis with significant variability in tumor type between adult and pediatric populations [31]. In the last few years, the increased use of neuroimaging has more frequently documented ventricular lesions in association with dilated ventricles and intracranial hypertension [12, 18]. Their deep location and proximity to eloquent neurovascular anatomy complicate surgical approach and resection. Even today, microsurgical removal is considered the best therapeutic option in most cases, but it is not without limitations. It remains challenging and is fraught with potential complications, which may be functional and cognitive or even life-threatening. Because of the central location of intra and para-ventricular tumors, commonly employed open surgical approaches have a relative increase in potential morbidity and mortality [6, 11, 33]. Furthermore, due to the poor outcome of these patients after the surgery, adjuvant chemotherapy and radiotherapy are not always possible. The need for a less invasive but equally effective surgical approach to intraventricular pathology has directed the attention of many in the neurosurgical community towards neuroendoscopy. Intraventricular tumors are ideal indications for neuroendoscopic surgery. In fact, because intraventricular tumors often obstruct CSF pathways, resulting in ventricular dilation, sufficient space for maneuvering with the endoscopes is available. Advantages of the endoscopic approach compared to microsurgical resection include greater visualization and illumination in the depth of the ventricles as well as less brain tissue damage and retraction. Craniotomies can be avoided because endoscopes are inserted through only one burr hole. Working through an operative sheath protects the surrounding structures such as the fornix, hypothalamus, and vessels. Neuroendoscopy is presently considered a minimally invasive surgical approach to expanding lesions bulging into the ventricle, as a relevant tool in performing biopsy procedures, discontinuation of cystic walls or tumor removal in selected cases [3, 8, 9, 22, 23]. As our experience had broadened, partial tumor resection was performed. Finally, it became possible to remove selected tumors completely with pure endoscopic technique [1, 26, 29]. However, the majority of data in the neurosurgical literature originate from studies on endoscopic colloid cyst resection [14,

30]. Data regarding endoscopic resection of other intraventricular tumors exist primarily in case reports and small series with insufficient sample size to draw meaningful conclusions. The evolution of high quality video in endoscopy associated with the introduction of the thulium (™) laser and the ultrasound aspirator has recently improved the neuroendoscopic procedures and report of tumor resection [5, 13, 16, 23, 24]. By revisiting our experience from 2002 to 2020, the goal of this chapter is to review the indications and the evolution of the neuroendoscopy in the treatment of ventricular tumors as an alternative to microsurgery and, in selected cases, in combination with chemotherapy and radiotherapy [7, 15, 27] and to provide a better understanding of this technique's virtues and limitations.

INSTITUTIONAL EXPERIENCE

From 2002 to 2020, ninety-six patients with solid or solid cystic tumors arising from the wall of the ventricles underwent neuroendoscopic procedures. These patients ranged in age from 8 to 79 years (median 55 yr.). There were 54 males and 42 females, including 8 children. All patients were symptomatic: 29 (30%) patients presented classical intracranial hypertension syndrome. The others presented focal neurological signs as well ataxic gate, cognitive disorders, headache with papilledema. The patients had a median preoperative Karnofsky performance score (KPS) of 55 (range 30-70). During the preoperative MRI tumors were located: 40 (42%) in the third ventricle, 37 (35%) in the lateral ventricle, 2 in the fourth ventricle, 6 into the Sylvian aqueduct, 8 in the brain stem, while 6 as leptomeningeal carcimoatosis dissemination. A ventricular dilation with hydrocephalus or obstruction of CSF flow in all cases was present. Depending on the location of the tumor and the ventricle size, a unilateral access (mainly right side) in all cases was performed. Only in 24 cases with the help of the neuronavigation (BRAINLab system, Germany) the endoscope trajectory was planned. To control intracranial hypertension, through rigid (25%) or flexible (75%) endoscope, septostomy or cystostomy or third ventriculostomy (ETV) or tumor resection were performed. To obtain a diagnosis for further oncological treatment, during the same endoscopic CSF relief, a tumor biopsy was carried out. The thulium (TM) diode pumped solid state (DPSS) laser (Revolix LISA laser products, Katlenburg, Germany) for shrinkage or ablation of thick tissue and hemostasis of high vascularized tumor was used [16, 24]. The ETV was performed in 68 patients with non-communicating hydrocephalus. In 6 LG astrocytoma, the ETV was the only definite surgical treatment. In 20 cystic tumors, cystostomy and marsupialisation into the ventricle solved the clinical intracranial hypertension syndrome due to a relevant mass effect. In 12 patients, neuroendoscopic relief of CSF pathways by septostomy associated with the Ommaya reservoir or one catheter shunt was possible. Removal was possible in 6 case colloid cysts and 5 cystic craniopharyngiomas by restoring CSF flow without adopting other procedures. After intracranial hypertension control, in patients with 28 malignant gliomas, 18 metastases or leptomeningeal carcinomatosis and 6 lymphomas were allowed to continue tumor adjuvant therapy ameliorating the quality of life. In 6 cystic central neurocytomas and 12 ependymomas subsequent microsurgical removal was achieved. Other tumors included PNET, pinealoblastoma, radionecrosis and epidermoid cyst, malignant teratoma, in which the immunohistology defined the subsequent personalized treatments.

INDICATIONS

If a tumor causes an obstruction of the CSF pathways generating enlargement of ventricles, a neuroendoscopic procedure can be hypothesized. The main goal is to achieve divert CSF in order to restore CSF circulation and resolve neurological symptoms due to intracranial hypertension. This is the first step towards treating intra or paraventricular tumors occluding the CSF pathways. Instead of using a simple ventriculostomy with external drainage (EVD) or a V-P shunt, any neuroendoscopic procedure is considered a safe and less invasive procedure with the advantage of obtaining the tumor specimen for histological diagnosis [3, 20, 22]. Tumor tissue sampling can be carried out on any tumor that is visible at the ventricular surface. During the same neuroendoscopic procedure, relieving CSF circulation to improve the neurologic state of the patient by septostomy or ETV or other ventricular fenestration can be performed [20, 23, 32]. A thorough preoperative radiological imaging study to understand anatomy distortion due to the tumor mass effect is critical. These radiology images can be mapped into the neuronavigation software for endoscopic neuronavigation. The sagittal and coronal T2 MRi are helpful in planning a correct ETV, it is not always feasible in the standard target like for instance when a tumor in the thalamus bulges into the third ventricle. After the histological evaluation, subsequent treatment can be planned. In case of low grade tumors, microsurgical removal can also be an option, too. In case of malignant tumors, by ameliorating the KPS of patients, adjuvant chemotherapy or conformational radiotherapy as "personalized medicine" can be scheduled [7, 27]. Furthermore, the ETV can be the only definite treatment for benign tumors such as tectal low grade astrocytoma [22]. Endoscopic treatment is the best option for cystic tumors or avascular solid tumors. A solid tumor should not exceed 2 cm in diameter. The endoscopic piecemeal removal may become time consuming and ineffective if the tumor is too large. Large cystic tumors can be reduced by fenestration or partial resection of the cystic wall, such as in the case of ventricular cystic craniopharyngiomas (Figure 1). A preoperative MRI helps to understand the consistency and vascularization of the ventricular tumor: extirpation of soft and avascular small tumors is easier and more rapid. In large and vascularized tumors, in which an endoscopic resection is not feasible, the best option is microsurgical or tubular endoscopic assisted removal. With a small keyhole approach and endoscope assisted microsurgical technique, an effective and minimally invasive tumor removal without extensive brain dissection as proposed by Perneczky is feasible [25]. Recently, an endoscopic technique has been described to remove intraventricular tumors using a transparent tube or conduit to approach the ventricle [21]. Given that there are no limitations in movement of the instruments due to the narrow working channel, the dexterity of the dissection is improved.

Neuroendoscopic Challenges in the Treatment ...

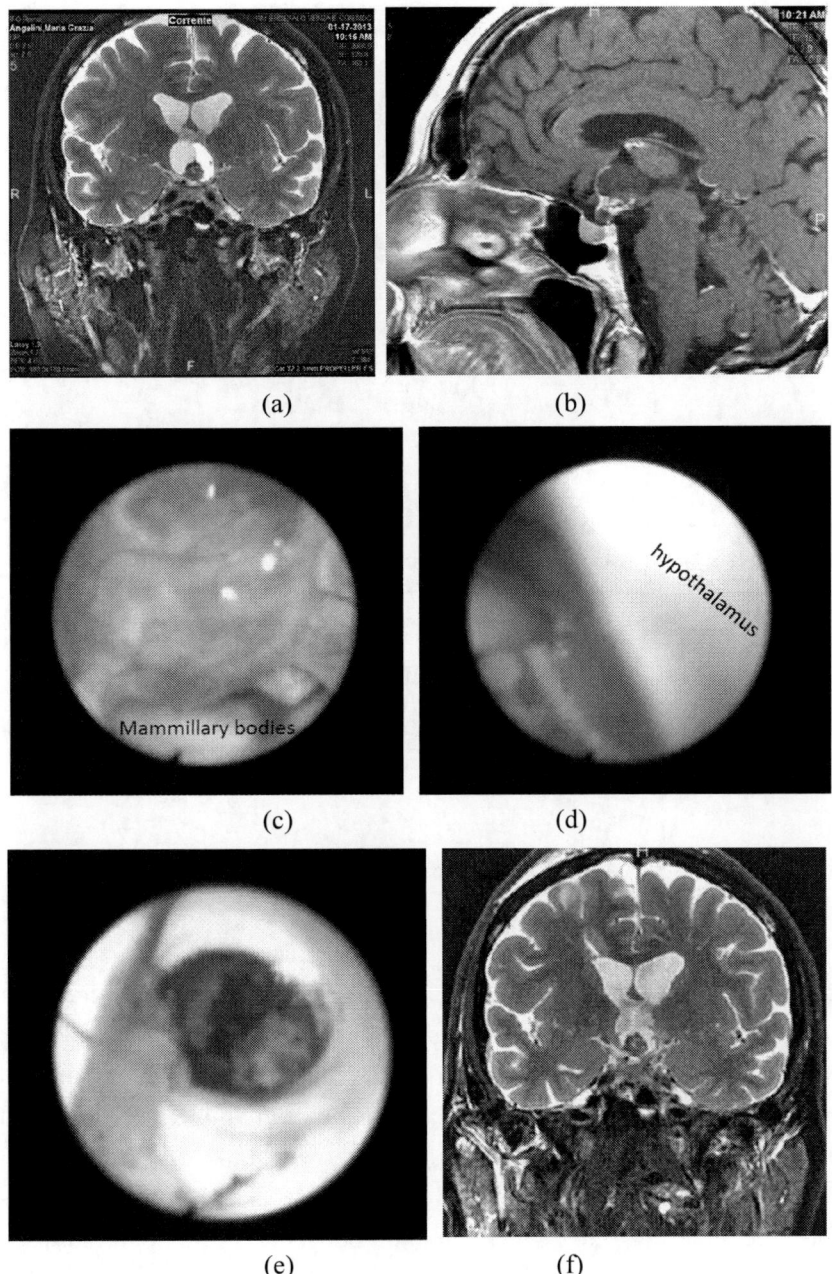

Figure 1. (Continued)

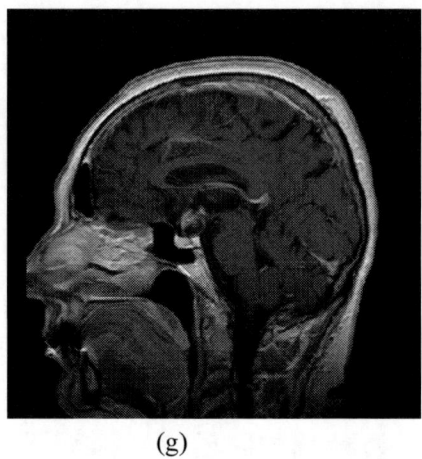

(g)

Figure 1. Third ventricle craniopharyngioma in 67 years old woman affected by intracranial hypertension: a) Preoperative coronal T2 MRi shows a tumor in the third ventricle consisting of two cystic components with the solid component partially calcified. b) Preoperative sagittal Gd T1 MRI shows the solid tumor overlying the floor of the third ventricle. c) Endoscopic view of the tumoral cyst through the foramen of Monro. d) Progressive ™laser shrinkage of the cystic wall close to the hypothalamus. e) Final view of the 3rd ventricle with craniopharyngioma calcified remnant. f) Six month postoperative T2 MRi shows the small solid remnant on the floor of the third ventricle without hydrocephalus and tumoral cyst. g) Six month postoperative Gd T1 MRi shows the calcified remnant on the tuber cinereum.

ENDOSCOPIC TECHNIQUE

The neuroendoscopic approach in ventricular tumors, always poses a challenge therefore surgical skills and high quality instruments are required. It is an advantage to use both flexible or rigid endoscopes associated with HD or 4K camera for exceptional magnification of the tumor-ependyma interface. To plan the entry point and follow the trajectory to the tumor of the endoscope, neuronavigation systems are mandatory, especially with rigid endoscopes, small ventricles and pathologic anatomy [20, 28]. A flexible endoscope allows safe navigation to look into hidden corners, but the narrow working channel limits instrument manipulation. Every procedure is time consuming, therefore a self-retraining holding device to hold the endoscope allows for a more comfortable working position with several instruments through the working channel. One of the major challenges comprises in ventricular tumor resection. In purely neuroendoscopic resection, the colloid cyst represents the typical tumor removal. In fact, these or similar tumors may be soft in consistency, whereas in others they can be fibrous and firm. In most of them, tissue removal is possible with a thin catheter for aspiration or grasping forceps and small scissors, however it is time consuming. A monopolar or bipolar diathermy probe or forceps are required for hemostasis, which are work better with a large working channel [26]. Alternatively, a microfiber laser, even inside the flexible scope, improves bleeding control while tissue cutting and vaporization is achieved at the same time, thus saving time. In our experience the ^{TM} laser for shrinkage or tissue desiccation of thick tissue and hemostasis of high vascularized tumor was used [23]. Currently, the ^{TM} laser is the only one that performs at low power achieving good efficacy both in hemostasis or tissue ablation in a liquid solution like in the CSF spaces. Recently, initial experience with ultrasonic aspirator (Sonoca, Sòring GmbH) in purely neuroendoscopic removal of intraventricular tumors has been reported [5, 13]. Currently, this instrument proved to be effective in complete resection of small intraventricular tumors, especially in cystic craniopharyngiomas or even calcified lesions. Partial resection of larger tumors was possible too. The disadvantage is that this instrument is still long and heavy and can be only introduced in the working channel of a Gaab endoscope (Karl Stortz GmbH). Gentle aspiration and continuous irrigation at low ultrasound energy is necessary in order to avoid ventricular collapse or excessive decreases in intraventricular pressure. Nevertheless, the strategy of a cystic tumor resection consists of wall opening and aspiration of contents, coagulation and complete wall removal. Finally, partial or total resection in piecemeal fashion is achieved to obtain valid histology as well as to restore CSF pathways. To avoid ventricular hemorrhage, feeding arteries and capsule vessels should be cauterized early by diathermy probe or laser. Because bleeding occurs frequently, continuous irrigation with lactated Ringer's solution at 37°C is performed to maintain a clear view and improve spontaneous hemostasis. It is ill advised to remove the endoscope in case of bleeding. It is best to leave it in place, rinse, and wait. A sufficient outflow of irrigation fluid should always be arranged to avoid a dangerous ICP increase.

POCEDURE-RELATED COMPLICATIONS

Severe complications resulting in mortality and permanent morbidity are fortunately very rare (0-3% in most reports in the literature) [1, 2, 26]. We had one death for intratumoral hemorrhage of a third ventricle vascularized malignant glioma. Intraoperative hemorrhage is the most frequently reported complication and thus a temporary EVD is requested. Other complications include memory deficits, hormonal disturbances subdural hematomas, CSF leaks and meningitis [2]. Nevertheless, the postoperative KPS improves with CSF relief, whereas tumor recurrence and survival are variable based on histology and subsequent treatments.

CONCLUSION

Ventricular tumors and related CSF pathway obstructions can be safely and effectively treated with neuroendoscopic procedures, consequently avoiding major surgical approaches and relevant post-operative morbidity due to its poor invasiveness. This surgical procedure is not limited to relieving non-communicating hydrocephalus, but is also useful for tumor removal, biopsies and evacuation of cystic lesions. In patients affected by malignant tumors, neuroendoscopy can be performed to control intracranial hypertension before starting adjuvant chemotherapy or radiotherapy. Small tumors may be totally or partially removed only via one burr hole and an endoscope, particularly by using the ^{TM} laser or the ultrasonic aspirator. In larger tumors, endoscopic-assisted microsurgery or tubular endoscopic-controlled resections are preferred over microsurgical instrumentation, thus avoiding lengthy procedures. Further experience and technological development may increase possible indications in the management of ventricular tumors in the near future.

REFERENCES

[1] Barber S. M., Rangel-Castilla L., Baskin D. (2013) Neuroendoscopic resection of intraventricular tumors: a systematic outcomes analysis. *Minim Invasive Surg.* 2013:898753. doi: https://10.1155/2013/898753.

[2] Bouras T. et al., (2013) Complications of Endoscopic *Third Ventriculostomy World Neurosurgery*, Volume 79, Issue 2, S22.e9 - S22.e12.

[3] Cappabianca P., Cinalli G., Gangemi M. (2008) Application of neuroendoscopy to intraventricular lesions. *Neurosurgery,* 62 suppl 2: SHC575 – SHC598.

[4] Chowdhry S. A., Cohen A. R. (2013) Intraventricular neuroendoscopy: complication avoidance and management. *World Neurosurg.* 2013 Feb;79(2 Suppl):S15.e1-10.

[5] Cinalli G., Imperato A., Mirone G., Di Martino G., Nicosia G., Ruggiero C., Aliberti F., Spennato P. (2017) Initial experience with endoscopic ultrasonic aspirator in purely neuroendoscopic removal of intraventricular tumors. *J Neurosurg Pediatr.* 19(3):325-332.

[6] Delfini R., Acqui M., Oppido P. A., Capone R., Santoro A., Ferrante L. (1991) Tumors of the lateral ventricles. *Neurosurg Rev.* 14(2):127-33.

[7] Ferreri A. J. M., Dell'Oro S., Foppoli M. (2006) MATILDE regimen followed by radiotherapy is an active strategy against primary CNS lymphomas. *Neurology,* 66: 1435-1438.

[8] Fiorindi A., Longatti P. (2008) A restricted neuroendoscopic approach for pathological diagnosis of intraventricular and paraventricular tumours. *Acta Neurochir* (Wien). 150(12):1235-9.

[9] Gangemi M., Mascari C., Maiuri F., (2007) Long-term outcome of endoscopic third ventriculostomy in obstructive hydrocephalus. *Minim Invasive Neurosurg.* 50: 265-269.
[10] Hellwig D., Grotenhuis J. A., Tirakoroi W., et al., (2005) Endoscopic third ventriculostomy for obstructive hydrocephalus. *Neurosurg. Rev.* 28: 1-34.
[11] Johnson R. R., Baehring J., Piepmeier J. (2003) Surgery for third ventricular tumors *Neurosurgery Quarterly* 13: 207-225.
[12] Koeller K. K., Sandberg G. D. (2002) *Cerebral intraventricular neoplasms: radiologic-pathologic correlation.* RG 22: 1473-1505.
[13] Ibáñez-Botella G., Segura M., De Miguel L., Ros B., Arráez M. Á. (2019) Purely neuroendoscopic resection of intraventricular tumors with an endoscopic ultrasonic aspirator. *Neurosurg Rev.* 42(4):973-982.
[14] Longatti P., Godano U., Gangemi M., Delitala A., Morace E., Genitori L., Alafaci C., Benvenuti L., Brunori A., Cereda C., Cipri S., Fiorindi A., Giordano F., Mascari C., Oppido P. A., Perin A., Tripodi M. (2006) Italian neuroendoscopy group. Cooperative study by the Italian neuroendoscopy group on the treatment of 61 colloid cysts. *Childs Nerv Syst.* Oct;22(10):1263-7. Epub 2006 Apr 29. Erratum in: Childs Nerv Syst. 2006 Oct;22(10):1375.
[15] Liu W., Fang Y., Cai B., Xu J., You C., Zhang H. (2012). Intracystic bleomycin for cystic craniopharyngiomas in children (Abriged Republication of Cochrane Systematic Review). *Neurosurgery.* 71(5):909-15. (doi: https://10.1227/NEU.0b013e31826d5c31).
[16] Ludwig H. C., Kruschat T., Knobloch T., Teichmann H. O., Rostasy K., Rohde V. (2007) First experience with a 2.0 micron near infrared laser system for neuroendoscopy. *Neurosurg. Rev.* 30: 195-201.
[17] Margetis K., Souweidane M. M. (2013) Endoscopic treatment of intraventricular cystic tumors. *World Neurosurg.* 2013 Feb;79(2 Suppl): S19.e1-11.
[18] Muly S., Liu S., Lee R., Nicolaou S., Rojas R., Khosa F. (2018) MRI of intracranial intraventricular lesions. *Clin Imaging.* 52:226-239.

[19] Najjar M. W., Azzam N. I., Baghdadi T. S., Turkmani A. H., Skaf G. (2010) Endoscopy in the management of intra-ventricular lesions: preliminary experience in the Middle East. *Clin Neurol Neurosurg.* 112 (1): 17-22.

[20] O'Brien D. F., Hayhurst C., Pizer B. et al., (2006) Outcomes in patients undergoing single trajectory endoscopic third ventriculostomy and endoscopic biopsy for midline tumors presenting with obstructive hydrocephalus. *J. Neurosurg.* (Suppl. Pediatrics), 105: 219-226.

[21] Okasha M., Ineson G., Pesic-Smith J., Surash S. (2020) Transcortical Approach to Deep-Seated Intraventricular and Intra-axial Tumors Using a Tubular Retractor System: A Technical Note and Review of the Literature. *J Neurol Surg A Cent Eur Neurosurg.* 2020 Dec 15. doi: https://10.1055/s-0040-1719025.

[22] Oppido P. A., Fiorindi A., Benvenuti L., Cattani F., Cipri S., Gangemi M., Godano U., Longatti P., Mascari C., Morace E., Tosatto L. (2011) Neuroendoscopic biopsy of ventricular tumors: a multicentric experience. *Neurosurg Focus.* 30(4): E2 (doi: https://10. 3171/2011.1.FOCUS10326).

[23] Oppido P. A. (2017) Endoscopic Reconstruction of CSF Pathways in Ventricular Tumors. *Acta Neurochir Suppl.*: 124:89-92. doi: https:// 10.1007/978-3-319-39546-3_14.

[24] Passacantilli E., Antonelli M., D'Amico A., Delfinis C. P., Anichini G., Lenzi J. et al., (2012) Neurosurgical applications of the 2 μm thulium laser: histological evaluation of meningiomas in comparison to bipolar forceps and ultrasonic aspirator. *Photomed Laser Surg.*;30(5):286-92.

[25] Perneczky A., Fries G. (1998): Endoscope–assisted brain surgery: part 1 – evolution, basic concept, and current technique. *Neurosurgery* 42:219-225.

[26] Schroeder H. W. (2013) Intraventricular tumors. *World Neurosurg.* Feb;79 (2 Suppl):S17.e15-9.

[27] Shono T., Natori Y., Morioka T. et al., (2007) Results of a long-term follow-up after neuroendoscopic biopsy procedure and third

ventriculostomy in patients with intracranial germinomas. *J. Neurosurg.* (3 Suppl. Pediatrics) 107: 193-198.
[28] Souweidane M. M. (2005) Endoscopic surgery for intraventricular brain tumors in patients without hydrocephalus. *Neurosurgery* 57:312-318.
[29] Souweidane M. M. and Luther N. (2006) Endoscopic resection of solid intraventricular brain tumors. *J. Neurosurg.* 105: 271-278.
[30] Tirakotai W., Hellwig D., Bertalanffy H. et al., (2007) The role of neuroendoscopy in the management of solid-cystic intra and periventricular tumours. *Childs Nerv Syst* 23: 653-658.
[31] Waldron J. S., Tihan T. (2003) Epidemiology and pathology of intraventricular tumors. *Neurosurg Clin N Am* 14: 469-482.
[32] Yamini B., Refai D., Rubin C. M. (2004) Initial endoscopic management of pineal region tumors and associated hydrocephalus: clinical series and literature review. *J. Neurosurg. (*Suppl. Pediatrics) 100: 437-441.
[33] Yasargil M. G., Abdulrauf S. I. (2008) Surgery of intraventricular tumors. *Neurosurgery* 62 (6) (SHC Suppl. 3): SHC 1029- SHC 1041.

EDITOR'S CONTACT INFORMATION

Soner Duru, MD
Professor of Neurosurgery
sonerduru@yahoo.com
Soner.Duru@cchmc.org

INDEX

#

3D CISS, 28, 46, 48, 50, 51, 52, 55, 56, 58, 61
3D SPACE T2, 46, 50, 51, 52, 55, 56, 57, 58

A

adenoma, 72, 77, 87, 89, 90, 91, 93, 94
adhesions, viii, 2, 6, 11, 28, 39, 49, 50, 51, 111, 112, 128
adults, 47, 52, 59, 62, 66, 71, 78, 79, 81, 87, 126, 139
age, x, 56, 61, 65, 67, 69, 70, 81, 86, 87, 88, 89, 91, 94, 107, 121, 127, 131, 134, 150
air embolism, 6, 18
anatomy, ix, x, 14, 22, 26, 28, 36, 47, 48, 51, 61, 63, 65, 79, 104, 123, 128, 133, 135, 139, 141, 149, 152, 154
angiofibroma, 88, 92, 93
astrocytoma, xii, 66, 111, 148, 151, 152
asymptomatic, x, 27, 53, 120, 130, 134

B

basilar artery, 47, 51, 123, 124, 128, 135
benign, vii, x, 52, 66, 74, 76, 78, 84, 86, 119, 120, 127, 143, 152
benign tumors, 152
bilateral, 5, 7, 9, 71, 126
biopsy, 86, 89, 148, 149, 151, 159
bleeding, 13, 55, 72, 108, 128, 155
blood, 18, 67, 68, 107, 128
blood transfusion, 68
blood vessels, 18
bobble-head doll syndrome, 28, 40, 138
brain, x, xi, xii, 26, 35, 46, 49, 55, 56, 57, 59, 61, 69, 76, 80, 90, 99, 103, 104, 107, 111, 113, 116, 123, 139, 141, 142, 147, 148, 149, 150, 152, 159, 160
brain tumor, x, xi, xii, 76, 90, 99, 103, 104, 107, 113, 116, 147, 148, 160
brainstem, ix, 25, 27, 28, 29, 30, 31, 70, 109, 111, 124, 128, 135
bulbar dysfunction, 27

C

catheter, xii, 29, 30, 31, 34, 35, 36, 38, 131, 135, 148, 151, 155
cerebrospinal fluid, vii, ix, x, xi, 25, 51, 52, 54, 59, 60, 63, 67, 100, 101, 119, 120, 143, 145, 147
chemotherapy, xii, 79, 85, 86, 148, 149, 152, 156
childhood, 61, 66, 69, 74, 76, 80, 90, 121, 143
children, ix, 40, 42, 43, 47, 49, 52, 59, 61, 62, 65, 66, 67, 68, 69, 70, 71, 72, 74, 75, 77, 78, 79, 80, 81, 84, 86, 87, 88, 89, 90, 91, 93, 94, 95, 96, 97, 98, 99, 100, 101, 102, 107, 111, 118, 121, 126, 132, 135, 138, 139, 140, 145, 150, 158
classification, xi, 63, 120, 124, 125, 130, 135, 138
communication, 47, 51, 59, 61, 63, 123, 146
complications, viii, ix, x, xii, 2, 6, 11, 13, 14, 31, 37, 46, 47, 51, 52, 53, 54, 55, 65, 67, 68, 74, 81, 84, 88, 91, 127, 130, 134, 148, 149, 156
compression, 27, 28, 47, 52, 55, 78, 79, 124, 125, 134, 135
corpus callosum, 49, 50, 61, 62, 121, 128
cranial nerve, 27, 52, 67, 71, 91, 109, 110, 111, 114, 126, 130
craniopharyngioma, 72, 75, 76, 87, 88, 89, 90, 91, 93, 94, 104, 105, 106, 107, 117, 154
craniotomy, xi, 39, 43, 53, 69, 81, 90, 107, 108, 120, 132
cyst, ix, xi, 39, 46, 52, 53, 54, 55, 57, 59, 60, 66, 72, 86, 93, 100, 120, 121, 122, 123, 124, 125, 126, 127, 131, 132, 133, 134, 135, 136, 137, 138, 139, 140, 141, 142, 143, 145, 146, 149, 154, 155
cyst ventriculostomy, 46

D

defects, 70, 81, 93, 94, 97, 98, 99, 101, 125
diabetes, 75, 87, 91, 127, 133
diabetes insipidus, 91, 127, 133
differential diagnosis, 52, 54, 127, 129, 149
diffusion, xi, 48, 52, 128, 147
dilation, 47, 124, 149, 150
displacement, ix, 25, 29, 57, 128, 135
drainage, 11, 26, 32, 81, 87, 89, 142, 151

E

edema, 29, 42, 47, 52, 112
electrocardiogram, 12
electrocautery, 22
electrolyte, 74, 90, 93, 94
electrolyte imbalance, 74, 90, 93, 94
endoscope, vii, viii, 9, 20, 29, 34, 37, 38, 68, 71, 98, 104, 105, 107, 108, 109, 111, 112, 113, 114, 115, 116, 133, 135, 139, 150, 152, 154, 156
endoscopic biopsy, 148, 159
endoscopic third ventriculostomy, vii, 46, 47, 60, 61, 62, 63, 148, 157, 158, 159
endoscopy, viii, 1, 6, 7, 12, 14, 39, 53, 130, 132, 141, 150
enlargement, 47, 121, 123, 125, 126, 134, 135, 151
epidermoid cyst, xii, 52, 109, 111, 148, 151
epilepsy, 3, 15, 80
equipment, 68, 70, 71, 95, 113, 114
excision, viii, 2, 9, 13, 15, 16, 53, 106, 108, 109, 110, 111, 112, 113, 114, 141
eye movement, 51, 113

F

fluid, 60, 93, 109, 122, 128, 140, 141, 144, 145, 156

foramen, 26, 28, 30, 34, 35, 39, 42, 47, 50, 63, 66, 72, 88, 124, 128, 132, 154
fourth ventriculostomy, 42, 46

G

ganglion, ix, 2, 4, 5, 7, 9, 10, 11, 14, 15, 17, 20, 21
growth, 66, 68, 69, 70, 77, 78, 81, 97, 100
growth hormone, 77
guidance, 21, 95, 108

H

headache, 92, 121, 126, 129, 135, 150
hemorrhage, 47, 52, 74, 75, 80, 90, 93, 94, 126, 155, 156
hemostasis, 107, 151, 155
histological examination, 12, 129
histology, 86, 155, 156
history, 22, 52, 59, 63, 86, 117, 121, 138, 144
hormone, 76, 87, 127
hydrocephalus, vii, viii, ix, x, xi, xii, 25, 26, 40, 41, 42, 43, 45, 46, 47, 50, 51, 52, 53, 55, 58, 59, 60, 61, 62, 74, 117, 120, 124, 125, 126, 128, 129, 130, 131, 134, 135, 138, 142, 143, 148, 150, 154, 156, 158, 159, 160
hyperhidrosis, 3, 4, 7, 8, 10, 12, 13, 14, 15, 16, 17, 18, 19, 20, 21, 22, 23, 24
hyperprolactinemia, 127
hypertension, xii, 86, 98, 129, 130, 138, 148, 149, 150, 151, 154, 156
hypothalamus, 51, 105, 106, 114, 117, 133, 149, 154

I

identification, 107, 109, 132, 134

incidence, 5, 10, 14, 22, 76, 109, 121
infants, 68, 74, 81, 95, 126, 141
infection, 53, 88, 92, 122, 131
interference, 28, 46, 55, 59, 60, 63
intervention, 48, 50, 54, 72, 94, 95
intracranial pressure, 27, 47, 74, 86, 126, 134
intraventricular fenestrations, v, 45, 46
isolated fourth ventricle, ix, 25, 26, 40, 41, 42

L

leakage, 72, 81, 87, 88, 89, 90, 91, 93, 94, 95, 130
learning, x, 20, 104, 107, 113, 117
lesions, viii, x, xi, xii, 16, 27, 50, 52, 63, 66, 68, 69, 70, 75, 76, 78, 80, 86, 88, 90, 91, 93, 98, 99, 100, 101, 102, 113, 119, 120, 124, 127, 129, 139, 142, 144, 145, 147, 148, 155, 156, 157, 158, 159

M

magnetic resonance, 59, 61, 62, 63, 69, 121, 141, 144
magnetic resonance imaging (MRI), 28, 30, 31, 37, 38, 46, 48, 49, 50, 51, 54, 57, 58, 59, 60, 61, 62, 63, 69, 70, 73, 76, 77, 82, 83, 84, 85, 106, 108, 110, 112, 121, 127, 128, 134, 135, 136, 141, 144, 150, 152, 154, 158
malignant teratoma, xii, 148, 151
malignant tumors, xii, 148, 152, 156
marsupialization, xii, 130, 132, 133, 148
mass, viii, xii, 27, 28, 53, 74, 108, 124, 125, 126, 130, 131, 148, 151, 152
medulloblastoma, 111, 112
membranes, 28, 38, 50, 52, 55, 120, 123
meningitis, 26, 87, 88, 90, 91, 130, 156

microscope, 104, 105, 108, 110, 113, 114, 116
morbidity, xi, xii, 39, 46, 53, 87, 88, 93, 94, 115, 120, 132, 135, 148, 149, 156
mortality, xi, 11, 13, 46, 53, 87, 90, 120, 135, 149, 156

N

nerve, 4, 5, 9, 12, 20, 21, 23, 67, 86, 88, 91, 92, 109, 126, 134
nervous system, 18, 63, 139
neuroendoscopy, vii, viii, x, xi, xii, 26, 32, 39, 53, 103, 105, 117, 147, 148, 149, 156, 157, 158, 160
neuroimaging, xi, 27, 32, 61, 143, 147, 149
neuronavigation, 26, 32, 37, 38, 39, 42, 70, 73, 108, 111, 135, 150, 152, 154
neurophysiology, 70, 97
neurosurgery, viii, 40, 59, 60, 61, 62, 63, 97, 104, 117, 139, 145

O

obstruction, x, xi, xii, 26, 28, 39, 48, 50, 52, 55, 57, 92, 119, 122, 129, 133, 147, 148, 150, 151
occlusion, 26, 128, 132, 133
oculomotor, 51, 105, 115
optic chiasm, 107, 128, 135
optic glioma, 83, 88
optic nerve, 66, 67, 70, 78, 83, 86, 88, 89, 98

P

pathology, 39, 63, 70, 72, 75, 78, 86, 87, 88, 89, 90, 91, 94, 95, 96, 149, 160
population, 52, 74, 79, 97, 99, 100, 101, 142

R

radiologic assessment, 46
radiotherapy, xii, 75, 79, 85, 148, 149, 152, 156, 157
reconstruction, 12, 23, 55, 80, 81, 87, 89, 90, 91, 95, 96, 97, 101
recurrence, 14, 75, 78, 86, 91, 92, 133, 136, 156
resection, xii, 5, 7, 11, 16, 17, 18, 67, 71, 75, 76, 77, 78, 83, 84, 87, 88, 89, 90, 91, 93, 94, 98, 100, 101, 105, 113, 114, 117, 133, 142, 148, 149, 151, 152, 155, 157, 158, 160
resolution, 42, 47, 51, 52, 55, 57, 116, 130, 131, 140
responsiveness, 123
reticular activating system, 28
rhinorrhea, 66, 74, 80, 81, 88, 89
risk, 51, 54, 67, 75, 78, 81, 94, 131, 132, 133

S

septum, 46, 49, 50, 51, 61, 62, 63, 72
septum pellucidum fenestration, 46, 50
showing, 30, 31, 35, 36, 37, 38, 52, 54, 106, 108, 110, 112, 128, 136
signs, xi, 27, 47, 49, 74, 120, 126, 128, 129, 134, 150
slit ventricle syndrome, 26, 27
stenosis, vii, 28, 32, 34, 47, 51, 52, 59, 60, 62, 63, 128, 132
stoma, 46, 48, 49, 51, 55, 56, 58, 135
structure, 28, 50, 52, 134, 141, 145
success rate, vii, xi, 49, 75, 78, 82, 94, 95, 120, 131, 132
suprasellar arachnoid cysts, vi, x, 59, 119, 121, 125, 127, 134, 138, 139, 140, 141, 142, 143, 144, 145
surgical intervention, ix, 25, 29, 75, 76, 80

surgical removal, 84
surgical technique, viii, 78
sympathectomy, 5, 6, 7, 8, 15, 16, 17, 18, 19, 20, 21, 22, 23, 24
sympathetic denervation, ix, 2, 3, 4, 7, 9, 10
sympathetic fibers, viii, 1, 4, 9
sympathetic system, viii, 1, 3, 14
symptoms, xi, 12, 27, 49, 53, 75, 78, 92, 120, 126, 129, 134, 139, 151
syndrome, viii, xii, 1, 2, 3, 4, 5, 11, 13, 14, 26, 27, 28, 40, 41, 51, 88, 126, 138, 148, 150

T

techniques, x, xii, 9, 31, 46, 48, 51, 62, 74, 80, 81, 90, 94, 95, 103, 104, 113, 114, 116, 117, 126, 132, 133, 148
technological developments, vii
thoracoscopy, ix, 2, 6, 7, 10, 18
tissue, viii, 55, 56, 82, 115, 116, 133, 149, 151, 152, 155
trajectory, 30, 31, 34, 37, 38, 108, 150, 154, 159

trauma, 2, 52, 80, 116, 121, 122, 126, 134, 135
treatment, ix, xi, xii, 3, 4, 16, 17, 19, 21, 22, 23, 25, 28, 29, 32, 35, 39, 40, 41, 45, 46, 49, 51, 53, 59, 60, 61, 62, 63, 68, 75, 76, 79, 80, 84, 99, 100, 120, 127, 130, 131, 132, 134, 135, 137, 138, 139, 140, 141, 142, 143, 144, 146, 148, 150, 151, 152, 158

V

valve, 29, 123, 131, 135, 141, 145
ventricle, ix, x, xi, xii, 25, 26, 27, 28, 29, 30, 31, 34, 35, 36, 37, 38, 39, 40, 41, 42, 43, 47, 48, 49, 50, 51, 52, 58, 111, 112, 117, 118, 120, 124, 125, 127, 132, 133, 135, 147, 148, 149, 150, 152, 154, 156
ventricular tumor, vi, 107, 108, 111, 147, 148, 149, 152, 154, 156, 158, 159
ventriculocystocisternotomy, xi, 120
ventriculoperitoneal shunt, xi, 29, 41, 120, 135
vessels, 11, 13, 14, 109, 126, 149, 155
vestibular schwannoma, 109